Tasty Keto Air Frye Cookbook

Quick and Easy Meat Recipes
For Busy People

Rudy Kent

© **Copyright 2020 - All rights reserved.**

The content contained within this book may not be reproduced, duplicated or transmitted without direct written permission from the author or the publisher.

Under no circumstances will any blame or legal responsibility be held against the publisher, or author, for any damages, reparation, or monetary loss due to the information contained within this book. Either directly or indirectly.

Legal Notice:

This book is copyright protected. This book is only for personal use. You cannot amend, distribute, sell, use, quote or paraphrase any part, or the content within this book, without the consent of the author or publisher.

Disclaimer Notice:

Please note the information contained within this document is for educational and entertainment purposes only. All effort has been executed to present accurate, up to date, and reliable, complete information. No warranties of any kind are declared or implied. Readers acknowledge that the author is not engaging in the rendering of legal, financial, medical or professional advice. The content within this book has been derived from various sources. Please consult a licensed professional before attempting any techniques outlined in this book.

By reading this document, the reader agrees that under no circumstances is the author responsible for any losses, direct or indirect, which are incurred as a result of the use of information contained within this document, including, but not limited to, — errors, omissions, or inaccuracies.

Introduction

What's the difference between an air fryer and deep fryer? Air fryers bake food at a high temperature with a high-powered fan, while deep fryers cook food in a vat of oil that has been heated up to a specific temperature. Both cook food quickly, but an air fryer requires practically zero preheat time while a deep fryer can take upwards of 10 minutes. Air fryers also require little to no oil and deep fryers require a lot that absorb into the food. Food comes out crispy and juicy in both appliances, but don't taste the same, usually because deep fried foods are coated in batter that cook differently in an air fryer vs a deep fryer. Battered foods needs to be sprayed with oil before cooking in an air fryer to help them color and get crispy, while the hot oil soaks into the batter in a deep fryer. Flour-based batters and wet batters don't cook well in an air fryer, but they come out very well in a deep fryer.

The ketogenic diet is one such example. The diet calls for a very small number of carbs to be eaten. This means food such as rice, pasta, and other starchy vegetables like potatoes are off the menu. Even relaxed versions of the keto diet minimize carbs to a large extent and this compromises the goals of many dieters. They end up having to exert large amounts of willpower to follow the diet. This doesn't do them any favors since willpower is like a muscle. At some point, it tires and this is when the dieter goes right back to their old pattern of eating. I have personal experience with this. In terms of health benefits, the keto diet offers the most. The reduction of carbs forces your body to mobilize fat and this results in automatic fat loss and better health.

Feel free to mix and match the recipes you see in here and play around with them. Eating is supposed to be fun! Unfortunately, we've associated fun eating with unhealthy food. This doesn't have to be the case. The air fryer, combined with the Mediterranean diet, will make your mealtimes fun-filled again and full of taste. There's no grease and messy cleanups to deal with anymore. Are you excited yet?

You should be! You're about to embark on a journey full of air fried goodness!

Table of Contents

Introduction 5

BBQ Meatloaf 9
Delicious Chicken Fajita Casserole 13
Simple & giusy Steack 15
Porck ChopFries 17
Spicy Pork Patties 17
Spicy Parmesan Pork Chops 19
Air Fried Pork Bites 21
Steak Tips 23
Ranch Patties 25
Easy Beef Kebabs 27
Air Fryer Beef Fajitas 29
Juicy Pork Tenderloin 31
Lemon Pepper Pork 32
Stuffed Pork Chops 35
Air Fryer Lamb Chops 37
Breaded Pork Chops 39
Creole Seasoned Pork Chops 41
Coconut Pork Chops 43
Jerk Pork Cubes 45
Smokey Steaks 47
Simple Beef Kabab 48
Spicy Pork Tenderloin 51
Garlic Thyme Lamb Chops 53
Delicious Herb Beef Patties 55
Roasted Sirloin Steak 57
Basil Cheese Lamb Patties 59

Air Fryer Stew Meat 61
Ranch Pork Chops 63
Taco Stuffed Peppers 65
Garlicky Pork Chops 67
Dijon Pork Chops 69
Pecan Dijon Pork Chops 71
Marinated Ribeye Steaks 73
Pork Kebabs 76
Herb Pork Chops 78
Pork Chops 80
Beef Kebabs 82
Rosemary Beef Tips 84
Sirloin Steak 86
Steak & Mushrooms 88
Flavorful Burger Patties 90
Baked Beef & Broccoli 92
Spiced Pork Tenderloin 94
Spicy Pork Chops 96
Lemon Herb Lamb Chops 98
Cajun Herb Pork Chops 100
Thai Pork Chops 102
Spicy Asian Lamb 103
Chipotle Steak 106

BBQ Meatloaf

Preparation Time:

10 minutes

Cooking Time:

35 minutes

Serve: 8

Ingredients:

1 egg
1 tsp chili powder
1 tsp garlic powder
1 tsp garlic, minced
1 tbsp onion, minced
2 lbs ground turkey
2 oz BBQ sauce, sugar-free
1 tsp ground mustard
1 cup cheddar cheese, shredded
1 tsp salt

Directions:

1. In a large bowl, combine together all ingredients then transfer to the greased casserole dish. Select Bake mode.

2. Set time to 35 minutes and temperature 400 F then press START.

3. The air fryer display will prompt you to ADD FOOD once the temperature is reached then place a casserole dish in the air fryer basket. Serve and enjoy.

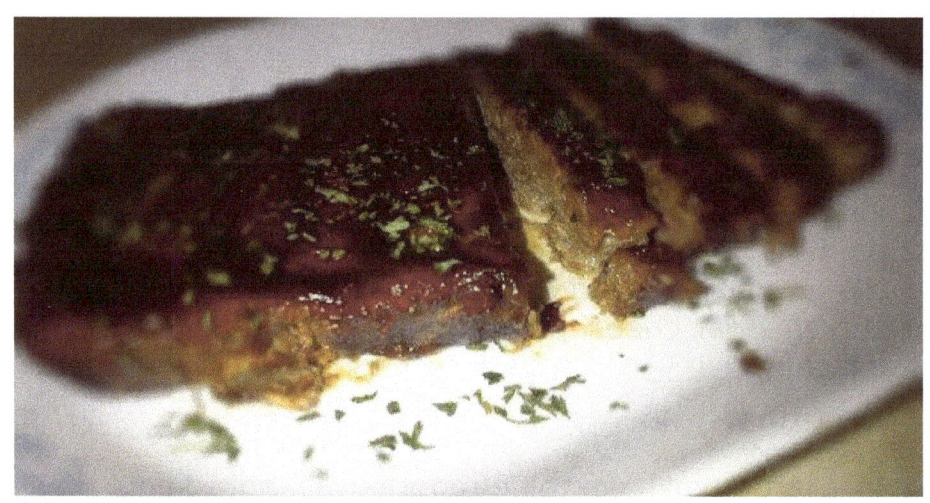

Delicious Chicken Fajita Casserole

Preparation Time:

10 minutes

Cooking Time:

15 minutes

Serve: 4

Ingredients:

1 lb cooked chicken, shredded
1 bell pepper, sliced
1/3 cup mayonnaise
7 oz cream cheese
7 oz cheese, shredded
2 tbsp tex-mix seasoning
1 onion, sliced
Pepper Salt

Directions:

1. Mix all ingredients except 2 oz shredded cheese in a greased baking dish. Spread remaining cheese on top. Select Bake mode.

2. Set time to 15 minutes and temperature 400 F then press START.

3.The air fryer display will prompt you to ADD FOOD once the temperature is reached then place the baking dish in the air fryer basket. Serve and enjoy.

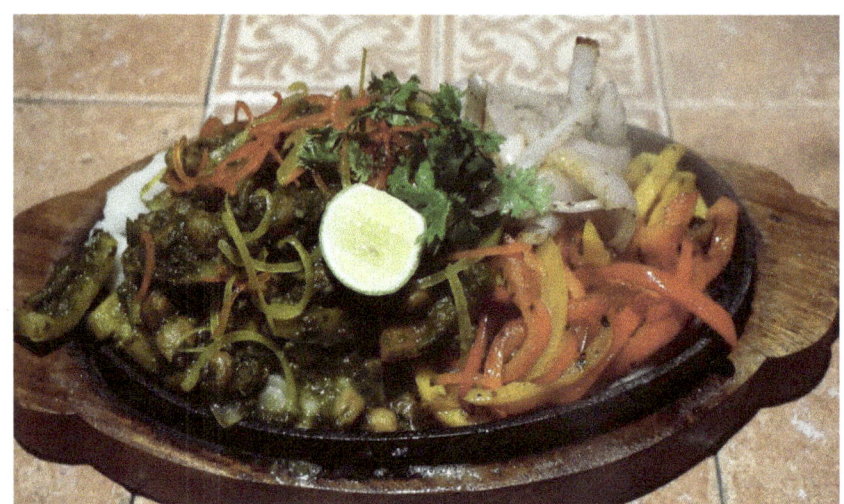

Simple & Juicy Steak

Preparation Time:

10 minutes

Cooking Time:

13 minutes

Serve: 2

Ingredients:

1.12 oz ribeye steak
1 tsp steak seasoning
1 tbsp olive oil
Pepper Salt

Directions:

1.Coat steak with oil and season with steak seasoning, pepper, and salt. Place the cooking tray in the air fryer basket. Select Air Fry mode.

2.Set time to 13 minutes and temperature 400 F then press START.

3.The air fryer display will prompt you to ADD FOOD once the temperature is reached then place steak in the air fryer basket. Serve and enjoy.

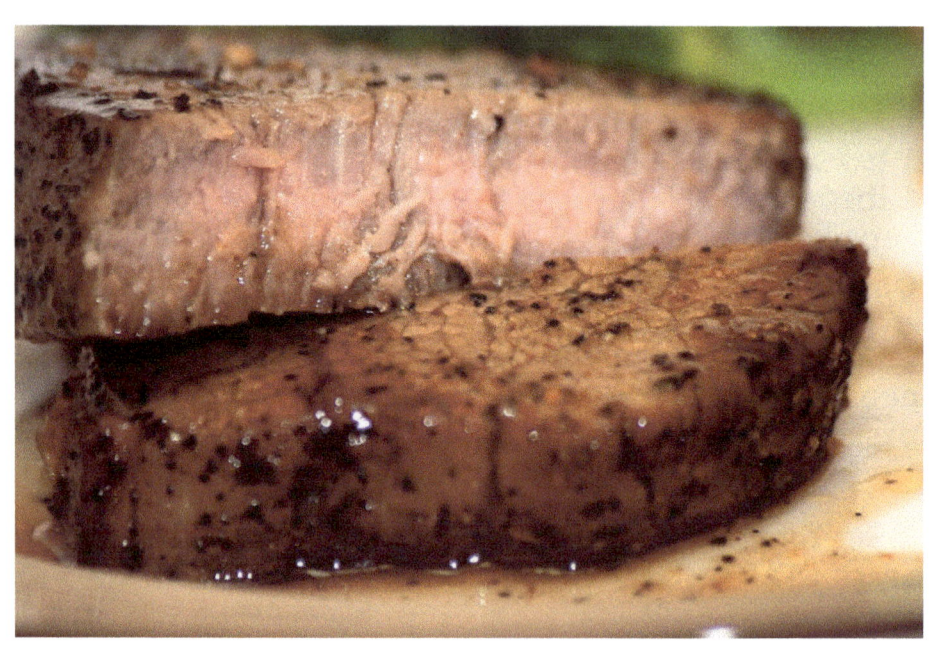

Pork Chop Fries

Preparation Time:

10 minutes

Cooking Time:

15 minutes

Serve: 4

Ingredients:

1lb pork chops, cut into fries
1/2 cup parmesan cheese, grated
3.5 oz pork rinds, crushed
1/2 cup ranch dressing
Pepper Salt

Directions:

1. In a shallow dish, mix together crushed pork rinds, parmesan cheese, pepper, and salt. Add pork chop pieces and ranch dressing into the zip-lock bag, seal bag, and shake well.

2. Remove pork chop pieces from zip-lock bag and coat with crushed pork rind mixture. Place the cooking tray in the air fryer basket.

3. Line air fryer basket with parchment paper. Select Bake mode.

4. Set time to 15 minutes and temperature 400 F then press START.

5.The air fryer display will prompt you to ADD FOOD once the temperature is reached then place breaded pork chop fries in the air fryer basket. Serve and enjoy.

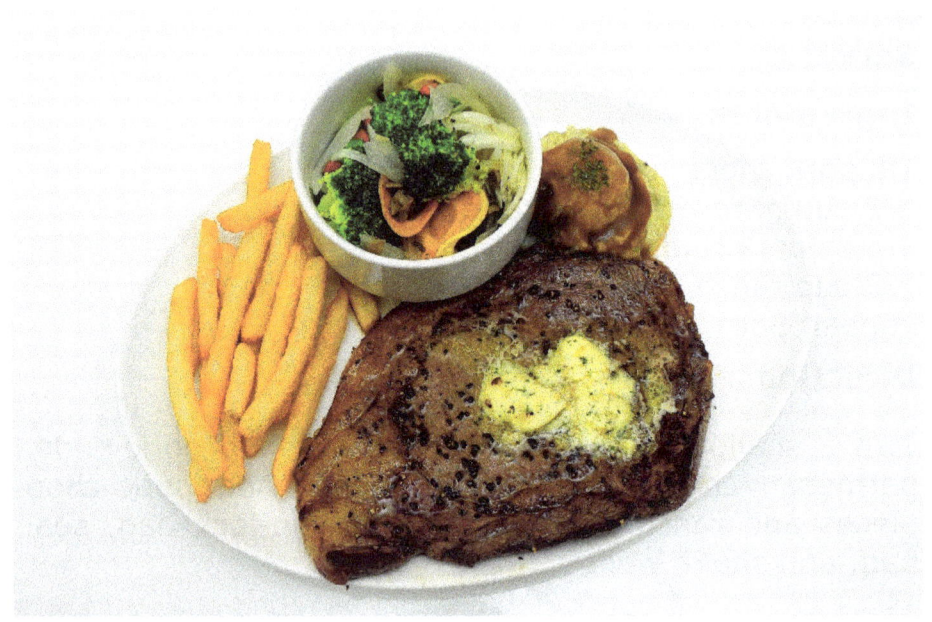

Spicy Pork Patties

Preparation Time:

10 minutes

Cooking Time:

10 minutes

Serve: 2

Ingredients:

1/2 lb ground pork
1 tbsp Cajun seasoning
1 egg, lightly beaten
1/2 cup almond flour
Pepper Salt

Directions:

1. Add all ingredients into the large bowl and mix until well combined.

2. Make two equal shapes of patties from the meat mixture. Select Air Fry mode. Set time to 10 minutes and temperature 360 F then press START.

3. The air fryer display will prompt you to ADD FOOD once the temperature is reached then place patties in the air fryer basket. Serve and enjoy.

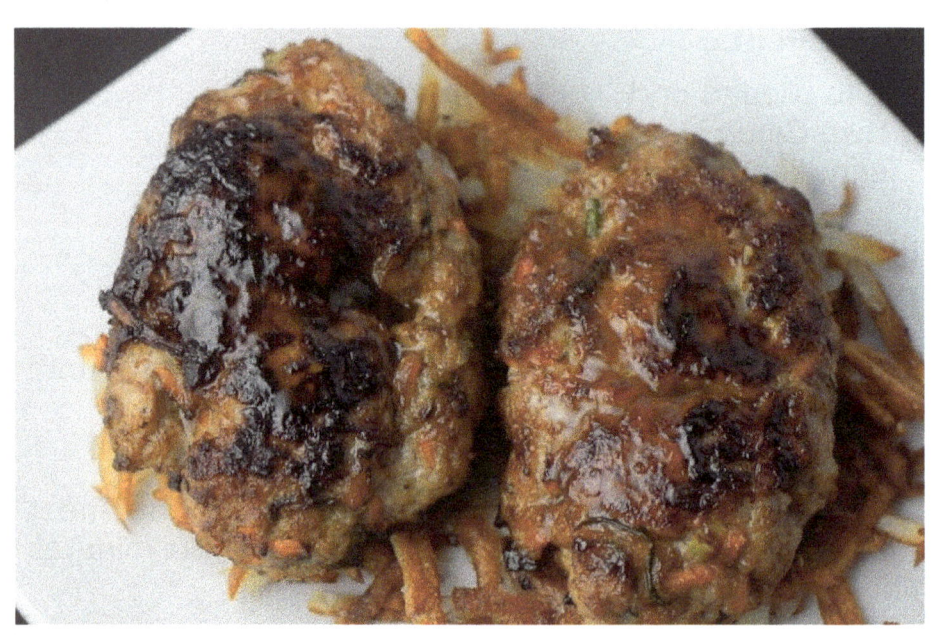

Spicy Parmesan Pork Chops

Preparation Time:

10 minutes

Cooking Time:

9 minutes

Serve: 2

Ingredients:

1 pork chops, boneless
1 tsp paprika
3 tbsp parmesan cheese, grated
1/3 cup almond flour
1 tsp Cajun seasoning
1 tsp dried mixed herbs

Directions:

1. In a shallow bowl, mix together parmesan cheese, almond flour, paprika, mixed herbs, and Cajun seasoning. Spray pork chops with cooking spray and coat with parmesan cheese.

2. Select Air Fry mode. Set time to 9 minutes and temperature 350 F then press START.

3. The air fryer display will prompt you to ADD FOOD once the temperature is reached then place breaded pork chops in the air fryer basket.

4. Turn pork chops halfway through. Serve and enjoy.

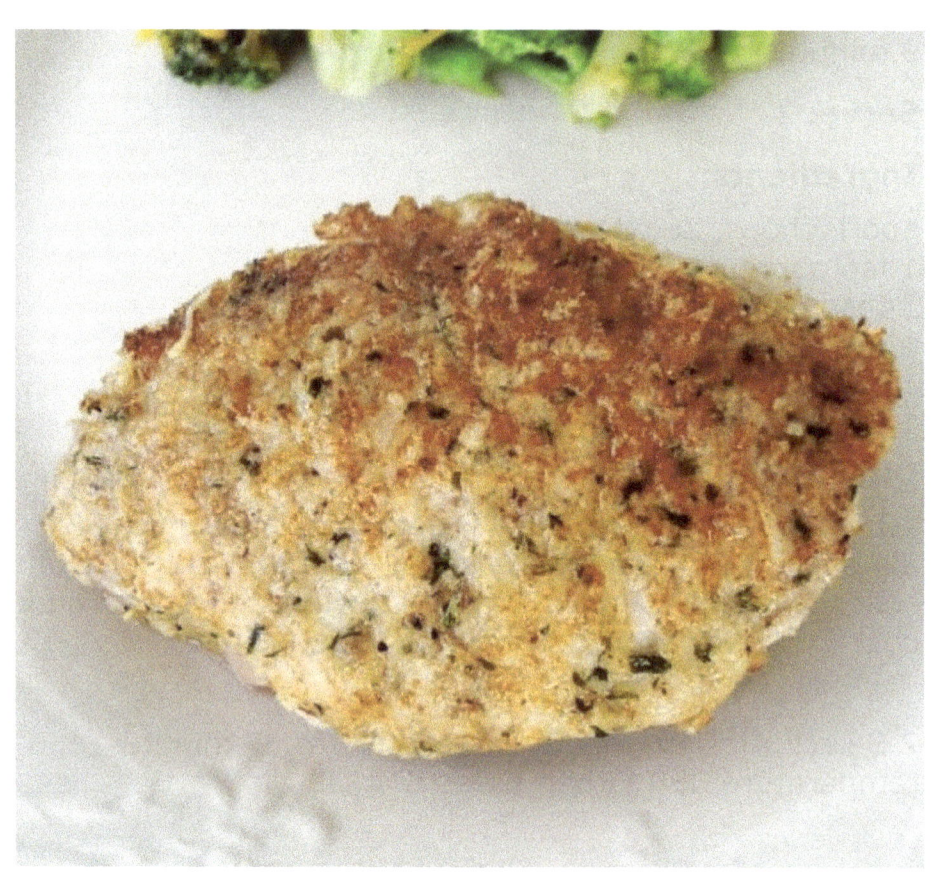

Air Fried Pork Bites

Preparation Time:

10 minutes

Cooking Time:

15 minutes

Serve: 4

Ingredients:

1 lb pork belly, cut into 1-inch cubes
1 tsp soy sauce
Pepper
Salt

Directions:

1. In a bowl, toss pork cubes with soy sauce, pepper, and salt. Select Air Fry mode.

2. Set time to 15 minutes and temperature 400 F then press START.

3. The air fryer display will prompt you to ADD FOOD once the temperature is reached then place pork cubes in the air fryer basket. Serve and enjoy.

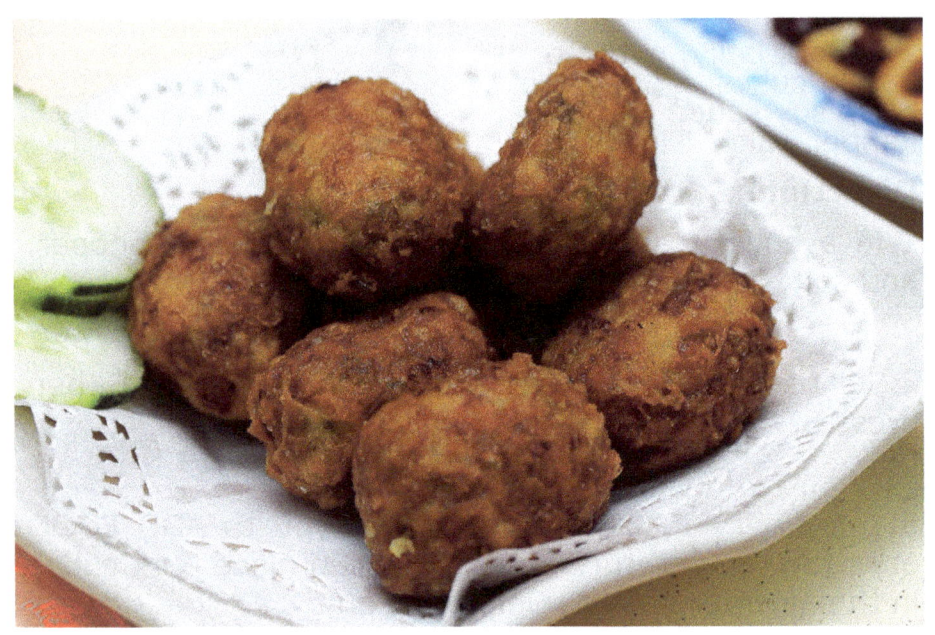

Steak Tips

Preparation Time:

10 minutes

Cooking Time:

5 minutes

Serve: 3

Ingredients:

1 lb steak, cut into cubes
1 tsp olive oil
1 tsp Montreal steak seasoning
Pepper Salt

Directions:

1. In a bowl, add steak cubes and remaining ingredients and toss well. Select Air Fry mode. Set time to 5 minutes and temperature 400 F then press START.

2. The air fryer display will prompt you to ADD FOOD once the temperature is reached then place steak cubes in the air fryer basket. Serve and enjoy.

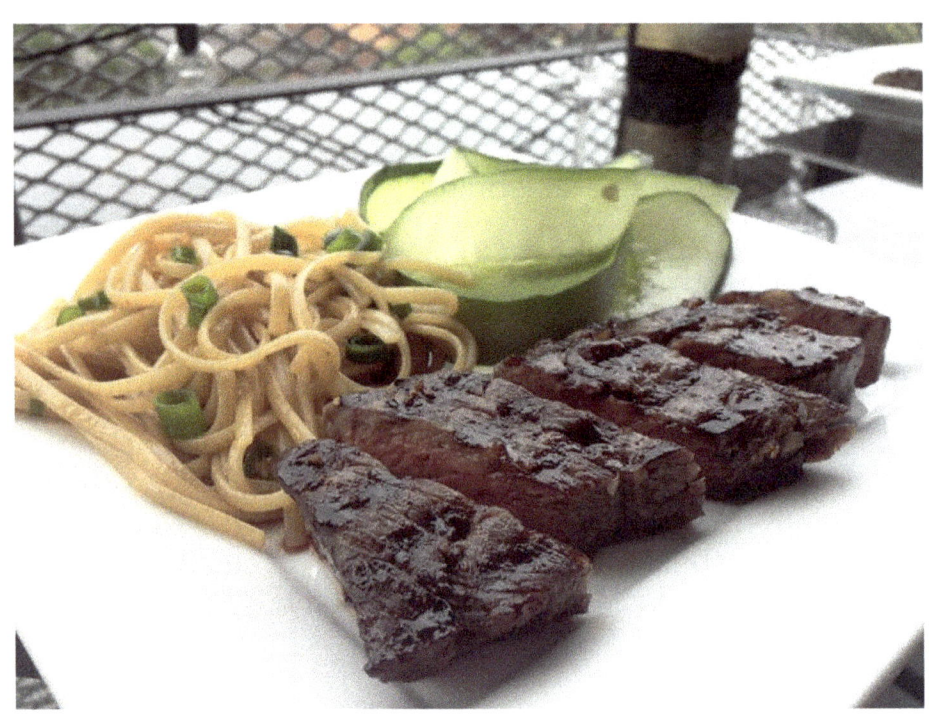

Ranch Patties

Preparation Time:

10 minutes

Cooking Time:

12 minutes

Serve: 4

Ingredients:

1 lb ground beef
1/2 tsp dried dill
1/2 tsp onion powder
1/2 tsp garlic powder
2 tsp dried parsley
1/8 tsp dried dill
1/2 tsp paprika
Pepper Salt

Directions:

1.Add all ingredients into the large bowl and mix until well combined.

2.Make 4 even shape patties from meat mixture. Select Air Fry mode. Set time to 12 minutes and temperature 350 F then press START.

3.The air fryer display will prompt you to ADD FOOD once the temperature is reached then place patties in the air fryer basket. Serve and enjoy.

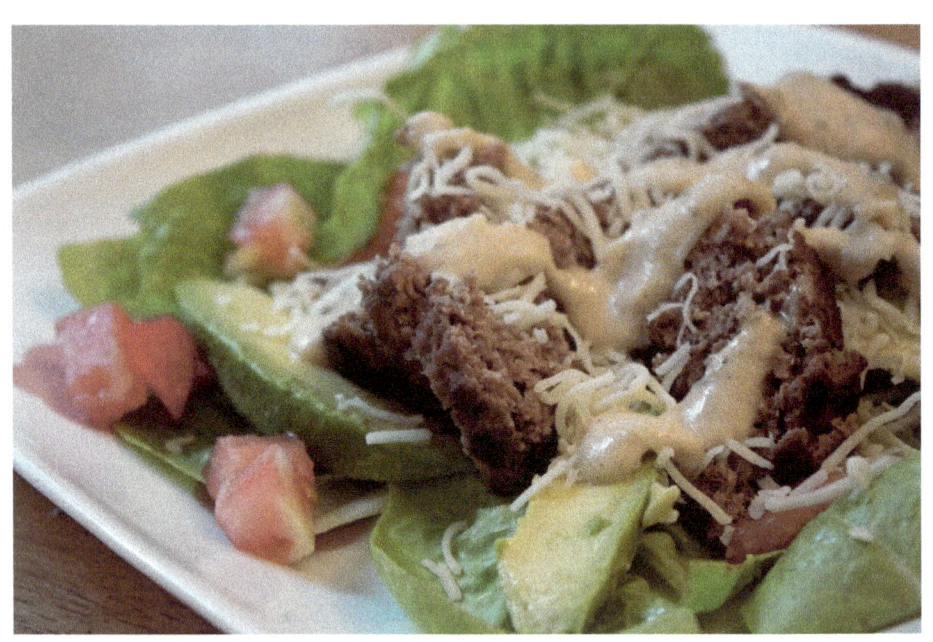

Easy Beef Kebabs

Preparation Time:

10 minutes

Cooking Time:

10 minutes

Serve: 4

Ingredients:

1 lb beef chuck ribs, cut into 1-inch pieces

1/2 onion, cut into 1-inch pieces

2 tbsp soy sauce

1/3 cup sour cream

1 bell pepper, cut into 1-inch pieces

Directions:

1. Add meat pieces, soy sauce, and sour cream into the mixing bowl and mix well. Cover bowl and place in the refrigerator overnight.

2. Thread marinated meat, onion, and bell peppers pieces onto the soaked wooden skewers. Select Air Fry mode. Set time to 10 minutes and temperature 400 F then press START.

3. The air fryer display will prompt you to ADD FOOD once the temperature is reached then place skewers in the air fryer basket. Turn halfway through. Serve and enjoy

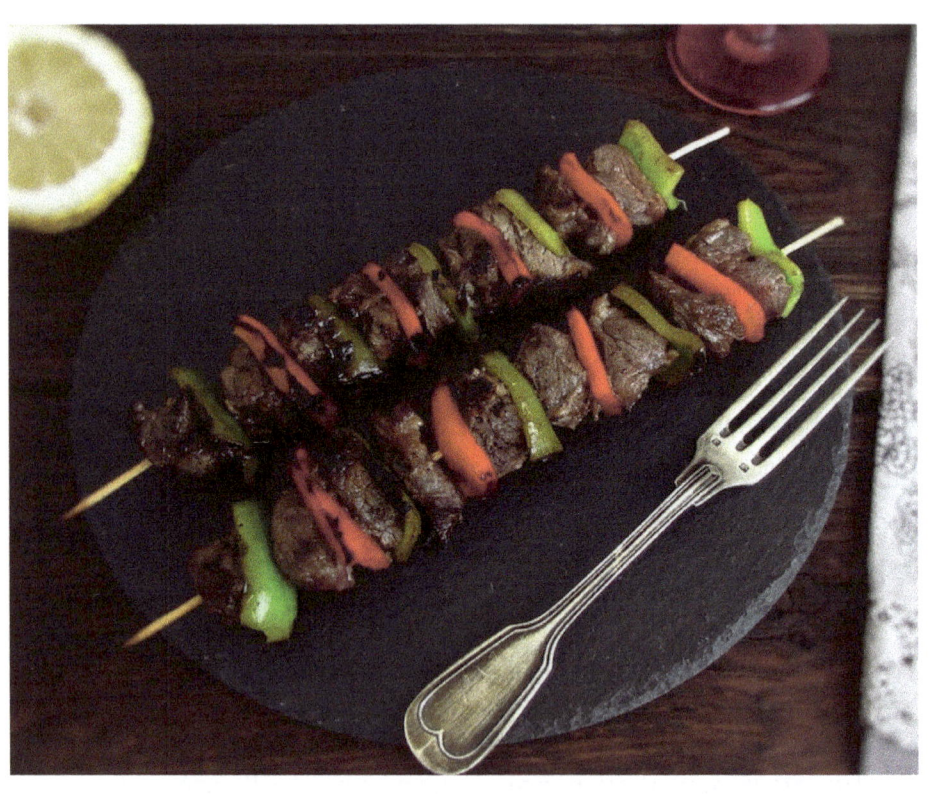

Air Fryer Beef Fajitas

Preparation Time:

10 minutes

Cooking Time:

8 minutes

Serve: 4

Ingredients:

1 lb steak, sliced
1/2 tbsp chili powder
3tbsp olive oil
2bell peppers, sliced
1tsp garlic powder
1tsp paprika
1tsp cumin
2Pepper Salt

Directions:

1.In a mixing bowl, toss sliced steak with remaining ingredients. Select Air Fry mode. Set time to 8 minutes and temperature 390 F then press START.

2.The air fryer display will prompt you to ADD FOOD once the temperature is reached then place fajitas in the air fryer basket. Serve and enjoy.

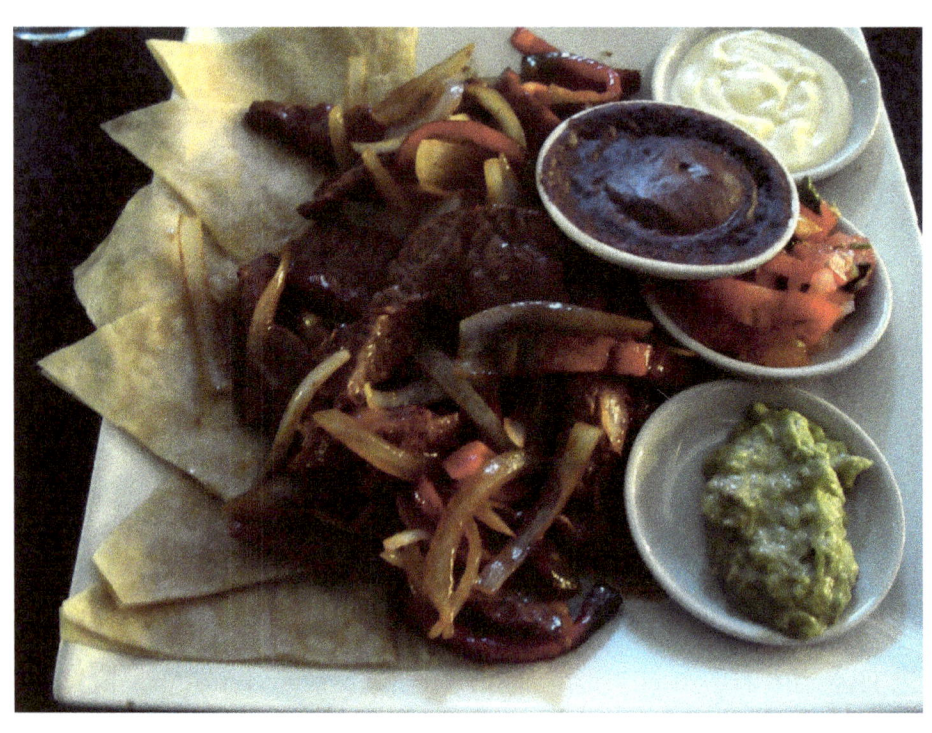

Juicy Pork Tenderloin

Preparation Time:

10 minutes

Cooking Time:

20 minutes

Serve: 4

Ingredients:

1 1/2 lbs pork tenderloin
2 tbsp olive oil
1 tsp garlic powder
1 tsp Italian seasoning
1/4 tsp pepper
1 tsp sea salt

Directions:

1. Rub pork tenderloin with 1 tablespoon of olive oil. Mix together garlic powder, Italian seasoning, pepper, and salt and rub over pork tenderloin.

2. Heat remaining oil in a pan over medium-high heat. Add pork tenderloin in hot oil and cook until brown Select Bake mode.

3. Set time to 15 minutes and temperature 400 F then press START.

4. The air fryer display will prompt you to ADD FOOD once the temperature is reached then place pork tenderloin in the air fryer basket. Serve and enjoy.

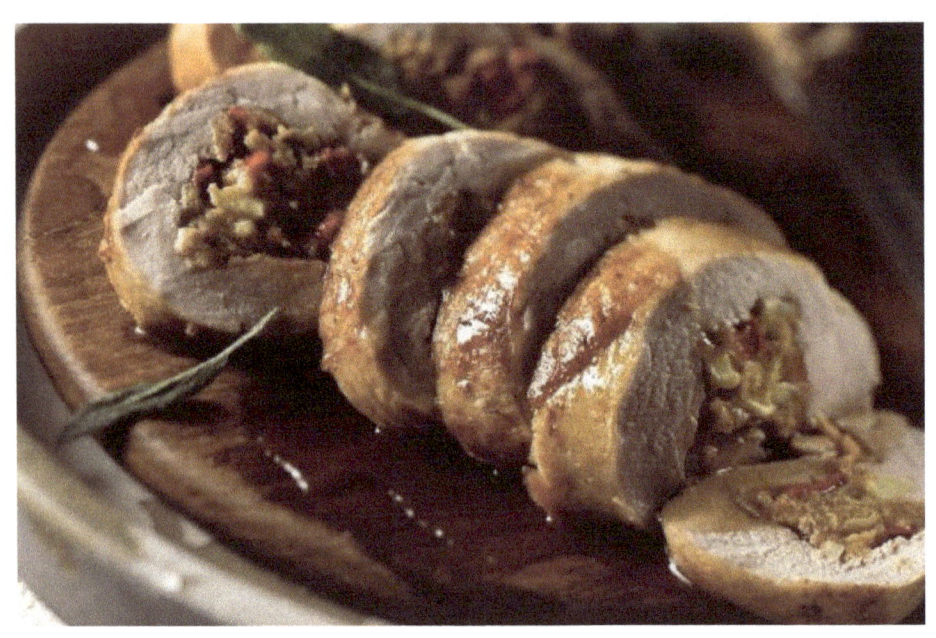

Lemon Pepper Pork

Preparation Time:

10 minutes

Cooking Time:

15 minutes

Serve: 4

Ingredients:

4 pork chops, boneless
1 tsp lemon pepper seasoning
Salt

Directions:

1. Season pork chops with lemon pepper seasoning, and salt. Select Air Fry mode.

2. Set time to 15 minutes and temperature 400 F then press START. The air fryer display will prompt you to ADD FOOD once the temperature is reached then place pork chops in the air fryer basket. Serve and enjoy.

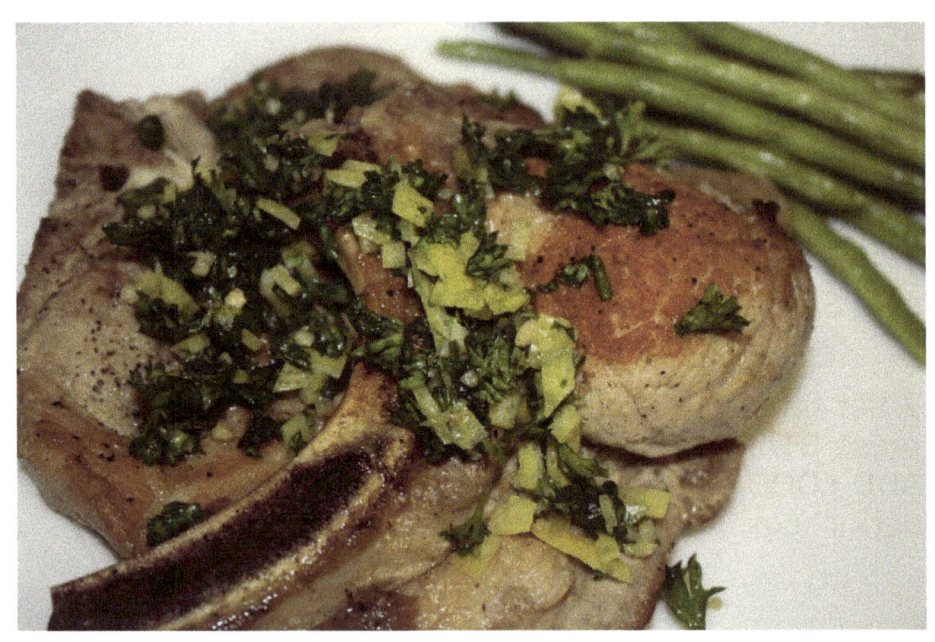

Stuffed Pork Chops

Preparation Time:

10 minutes

Cooking Time:

35 minutes

Serve: 4

Ingredients:

4 pork chops, boneless and thick-cut
2 tbsp olives, chopped
2 tbsp sun-dried tomatoes, chopped
1/2 cup feta cheese, crumbled
2 garlic cloves, minced
2 tbsp fresh parsley, chopped

Directions:

1. In a bowl, combine together feta cheese, garlic, parsley, olives, and sun-dried tomatoes. Stuff cheese mixture all the pork chops.

2. Season pork chops with pepper and salt. Select Bake mode. Set time to 35 minutes and temperature 375 F then press START.

3. The air fryer display will prompt you to ADD FOOD once the temperature is reached then place stuffed pork chops in the air fryer basket. Serve and enjoy

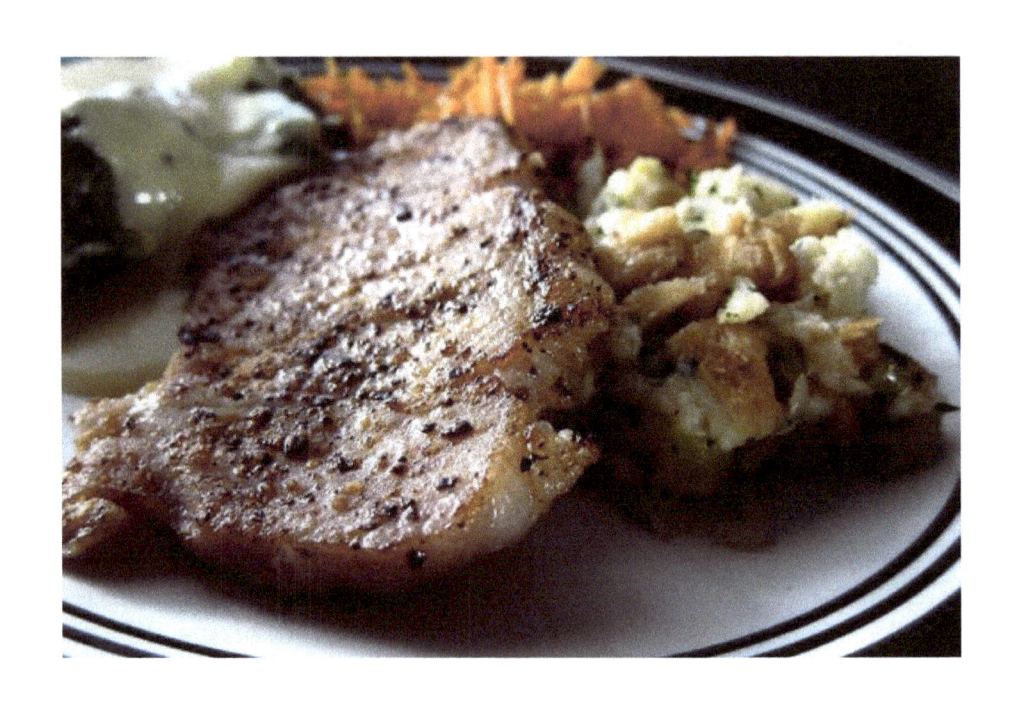

Air Fryer Lamb Chops

Preparation Time:

10 minutes

Cooking Time:

12 minutes

Serve: 4

Ingredients:

4 lamb chops
2 garlic clove, minced
3 tbsp olive oil
Pepper Salt

Directions:

1.In a small bowl, mix together thyme and oil. Season lamb chops with pepper and salt and rubs with thyme mixture. Select Air Fry mode.

2.Set time to 12 minutes and temperature 400 F then press START. The air fryer display will prompt you to ADD FOOD once the temperature is reached then place lamb chops in the air fryer basket.

3.Turn halfway through. Serve and enjoy.

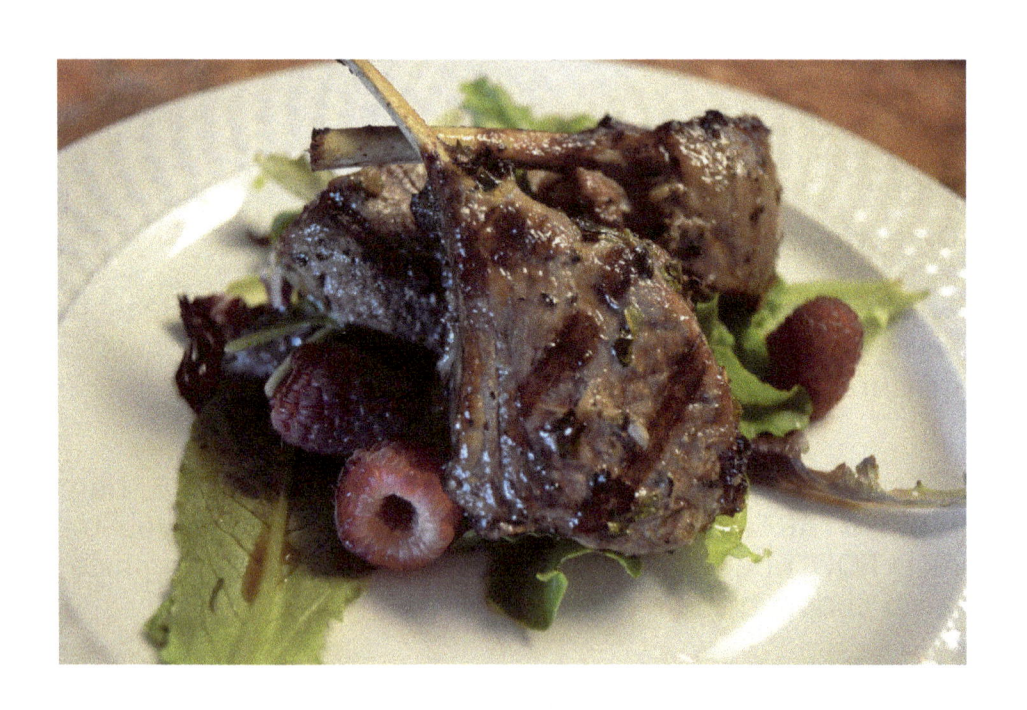

Breaded Pork Chops

Preparation Time:

10 minutes

Cooking Time:

20 **minutes**

Serve: 4

Ingredients:

4 pork chops, boneless
1/4 cup parmesan cheese, grated
1 cup almond meal
1/2 tbsp black pepper
1 tbsp onion powder
1 tbsp garlic powder
2 eggs, lightly beaten
1/2 tsp sea salt

Directions:

1. In a bowl, mix together almond meal, parmesan cheese, onion powder, garlic powder, pepper, and salt. Whisk eggs in a shallow dish.

2. Dip pork chops into the egg then coat with almond meal mixture. Select Air Fry mode.

3. Set time to 20 minutes and temperature 350 F then press START.

4. The air fryer display will prompt you to ADD FOOD once the temperature is reached then place breaded pork chops in the air fryer basket.

5.Turn pork chops halfway through. Serve and enjoy

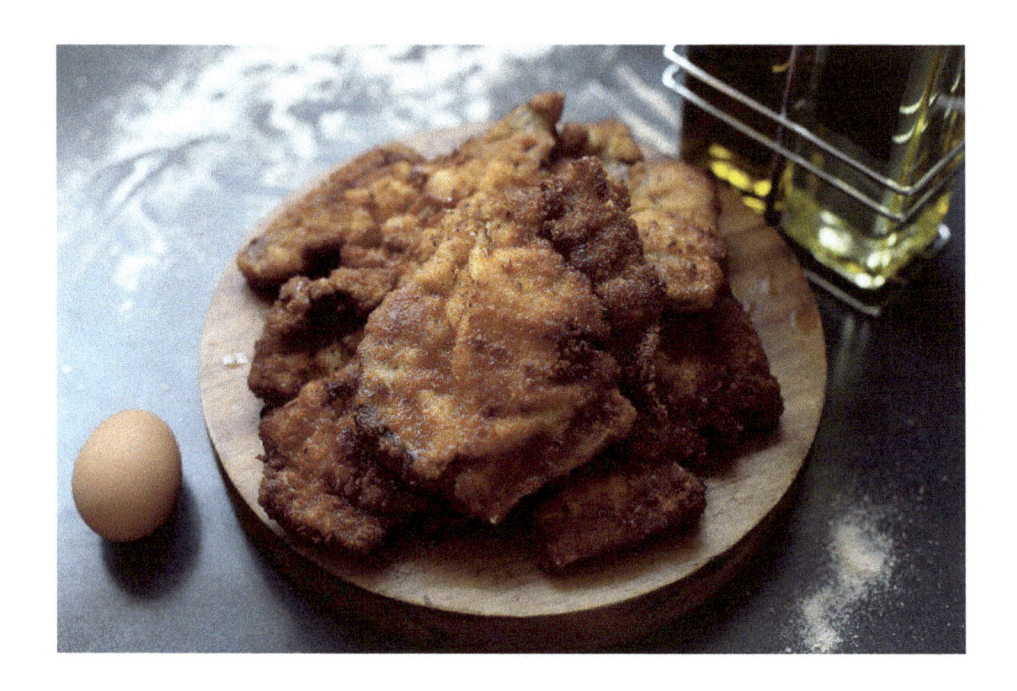

Creole Seasoned Pork Chops

Preparation Time:

10 minutes

Cooking Time:

12 minutes

Serve: 6

Ingredients:

1 1/2 lbs pork chops, boneless
1/4 cup parmesan cheese, grated
1/3 cup almond flour
1 tsp paprika
1 tsp Creole seasoning
1 tsp garlic powder

Directions:

1. Add all ingredients except pork chops into the zip-lock bag. Add pork chops into the bag. Seal bag and shake well.

2. Remove pork chops from the zip-lock bag. Select Air Fry mode. Set time to 12 minutes and temperature 360 F then press START.

3. The air fryer display will prompt you to ADD FOOD once the temperature is reached then place pork chops in the air fryer basket. Serve and enjoy.

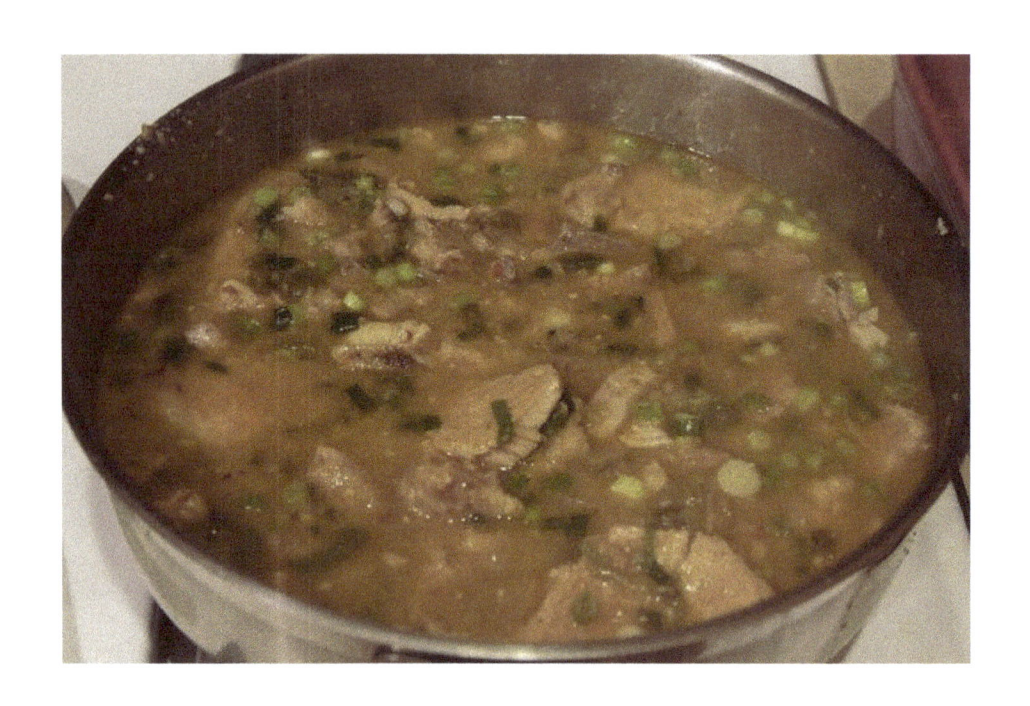

Coconut Pork Chops

Preparation Time:

10 minutes

Cooking Time:

14 minutes

Serve: 4

Ingredients:

4 pork chops
1 tbsp coconut oil
1 tbsp coconut butter
2 tsp parsley
2 tsp garlic, grated
Pepper Salt

Directions:

1.In a large bowl, mix together with seasonings, garlic, butter, and coconut oil. Add pork chops to the bowl and mix well.

2.Place in refrigerator overnight. Select Air Fry mode. Set time to 14 minutes and temperature 350 F then press START.

3.The air fryer display will prompt you to ADD FOOD once the temperature is reached then place marinated pork chops in the air fryer basket. Turn pork chops halfway through. Serve and enjoy.

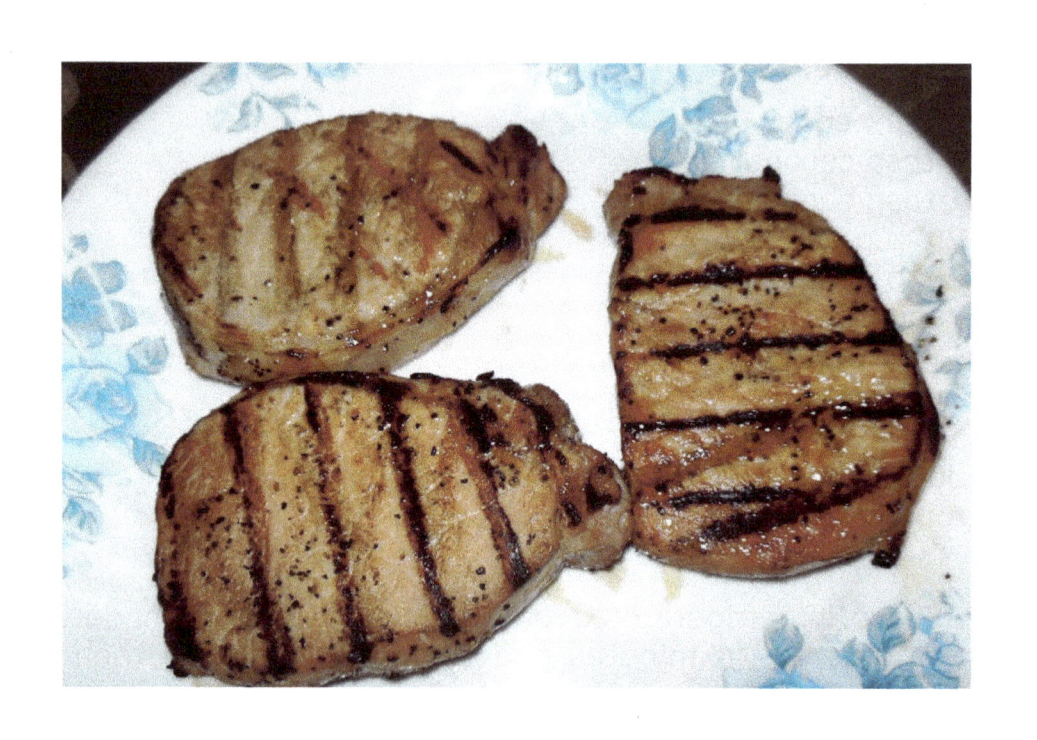

Jerk Pork Cubes

Preparation Time:

10 minutes

Cooking Time:

20 minutes

Serve: 4

Ingredients:

1 1/2 lbs pork butt, cut into pieces
1/4 cup jerk paste
Pepper Salt

Directions:

1. Add meat and jerk paste into the bowl and mix well and place in refrigerator overnight.

2. Select Air Fry mode. Set time to 20 minutes and temperature 390 F then press START.

3. The air fryer display will prompt you to ADD FOOD once the temperature is reached then place marinated pork pieces in the air fryer basket.

4. Stir halfway through. Serve and enjoy.

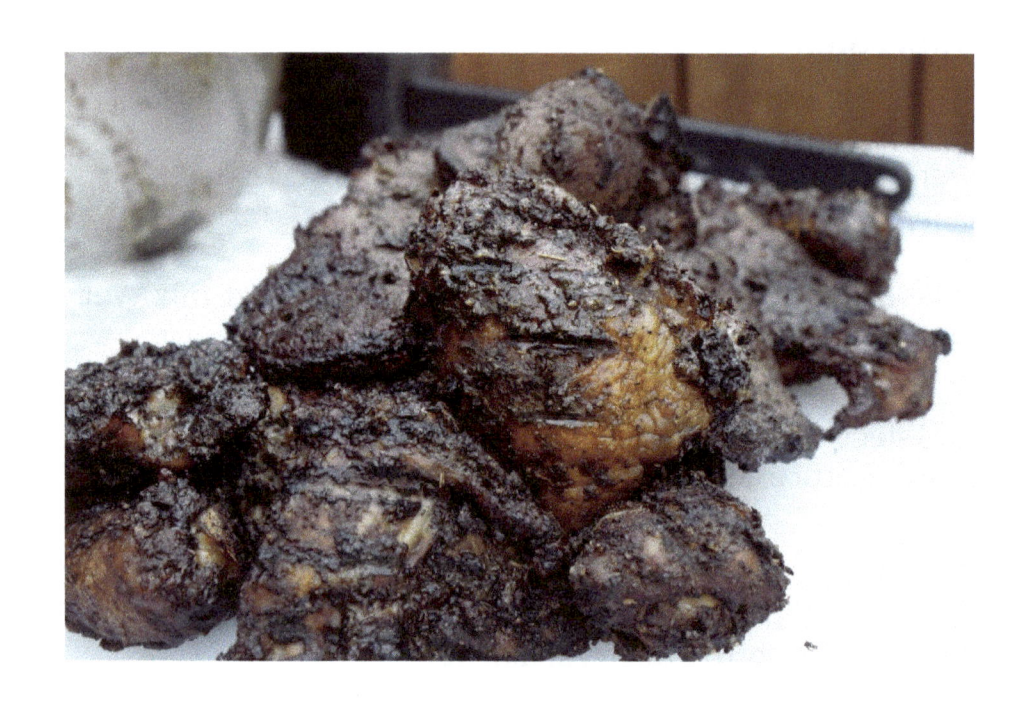

Smokey Steaks

Preparation Time:

10 minutes

Cooking Time:

7 minutes

Serve: 2

Ingredients:

12 oz steaks
1 tbsp Montreal steak seasoning
1 tsp liquid smoke
1 tbsp soy sauce
1/2 tbsp cocoa powder
Pepper Salt

Directions:

1.Add steak, liquid smoke, soy sauce, and steak seasonings into the large zip-lock bag. Shake well and place it in the refrigerator overnight.

2.Select Air Fry mode. Set time to 7 minutes and temperature 375 F then press START.

3.The air fryer display will prompt you to ADD FOOD once the temperature is reached then place steaks in the air fryer basket. Turn steaks after 5 minutes. Serve and enjoy.

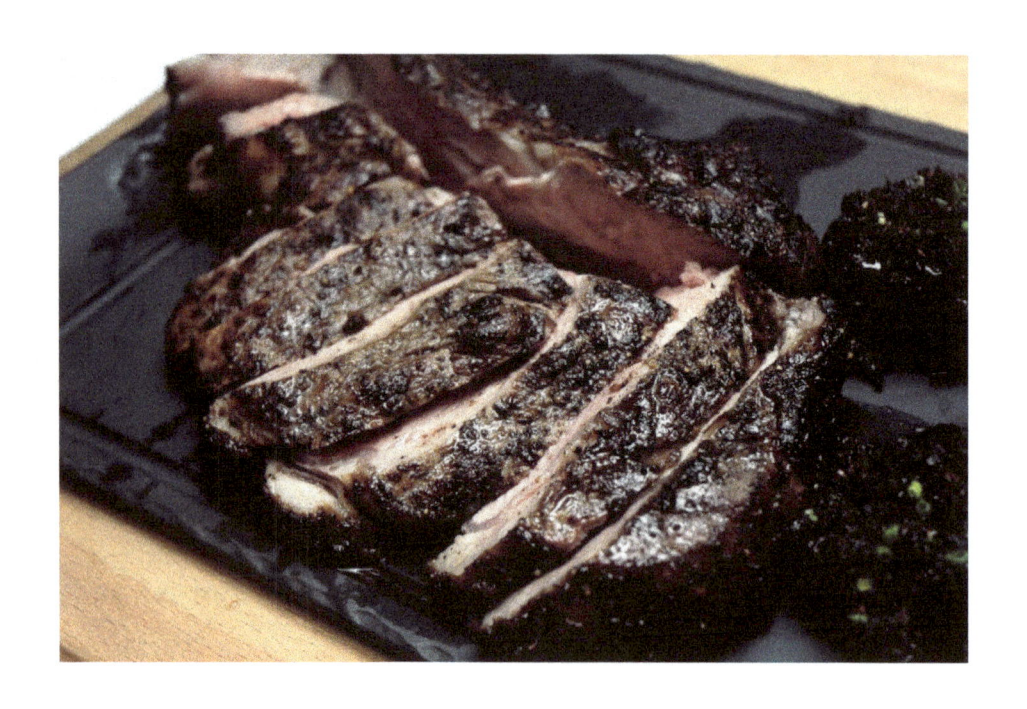

Simple Beef Kabab

Preparation Time:

10 minutes

Cooking Time:

10 minutes

Serve: 4

Ingredients:

1lb ground beef
2 tbsp kabab spice mix
1 tbsp garlic, minced
1 tbsp olive oil
1 tsp salt

Directions:

1. Add all ingredients into the mixing bowl and mix until well combined.

2. Place in refrigerator for 30 minutes. Divide mixture into the 4 equal portions and make sausage shape kabab.

3. Select Air Fry mode. Set time to 10 minutes and temperature 370 F then press START.

4. The air fryer display will prompt you to ADD FOOD once the temperature is reached then place kabab in the air fryer basket. Serve and enjoy.

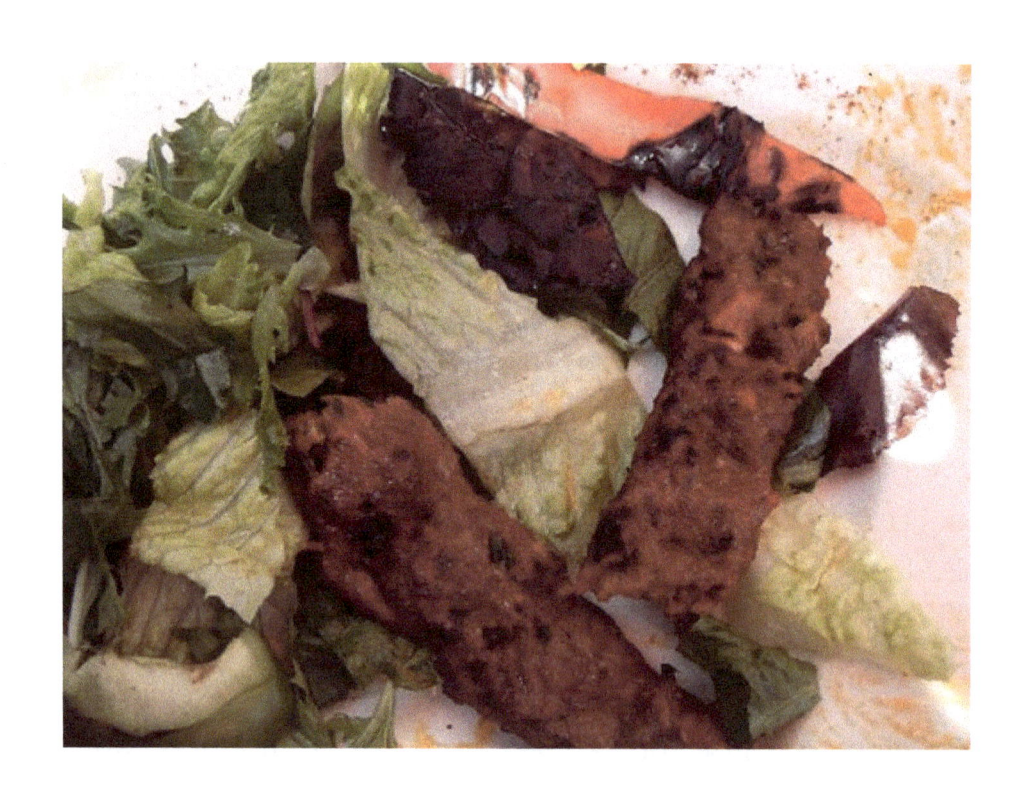

Spicy Pork Tenderloin

Preparation Time:

10 minutes

Cooking Time:

35 minutes

Serve: 6

Ingredients:

1 pork tenderloin
For rub:
1 tbsp smoked paprika
1 tbsp garlic powder
1 tbsp onion powder
1/2 tbsp salt

Directions:

1. In a small bowl, combine together all rub ingredients. Coat pork tenderloin with the rub. Heat ovenproof pan over medium-high heat.

2. Spray pan with cooking spray. Sear pork on all sides until lightly golden brown. Select Bake mode. Set time to 30 minutes and temperature 400 F then press START.

3. The air fryer display will prompt you to ADD FOOD once the temperature is reached then place pork tenderloin in the air fryer basket. Serve and enjoy.

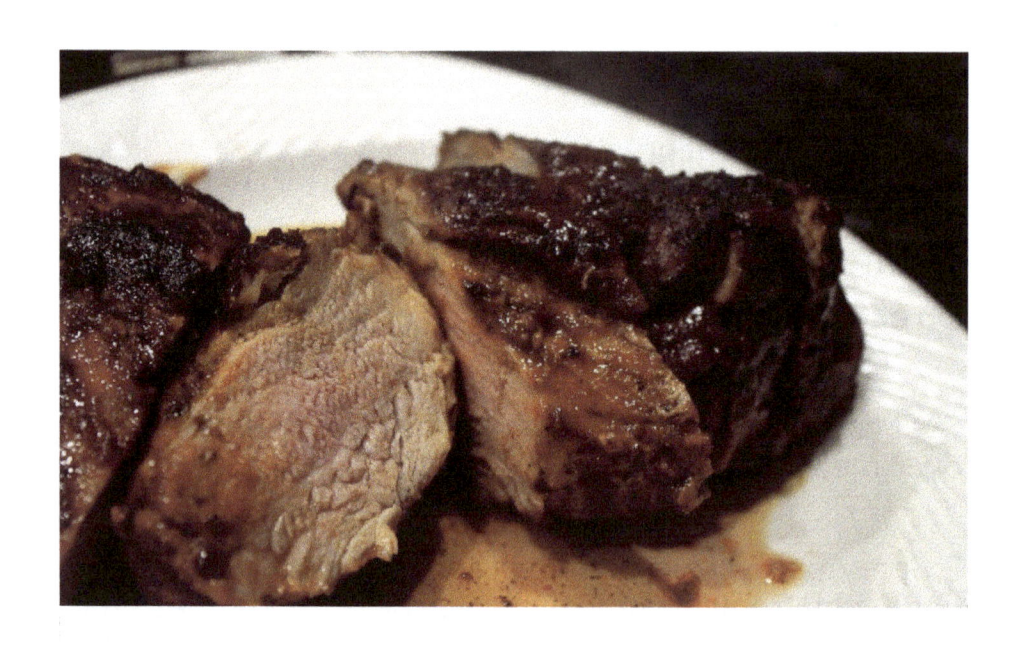

Garlic Thyme Lamb Chops

Preparation Time:

5 minutes

Cooking Time:

12 minutes

Serve: 4

Ingredients:

4 lamb chops
4 garlic clove, minced
3 tbsp olive oil
Pepper Salt

Directions:

1. In a small bowl, mix together oil and garlic. Season lamb chops with pepper and salt and rubs with oil and garlic mixture.

2. Select Bake mode. Set time to 12 minutes and temperature 400 F then press START.

3. The air fryer display will prompt you to ADD FOOD once the temperature is reached then place lamb chops in the air fryer basket.

4. Turn lamb chops halfway through. Serve and enjoy.

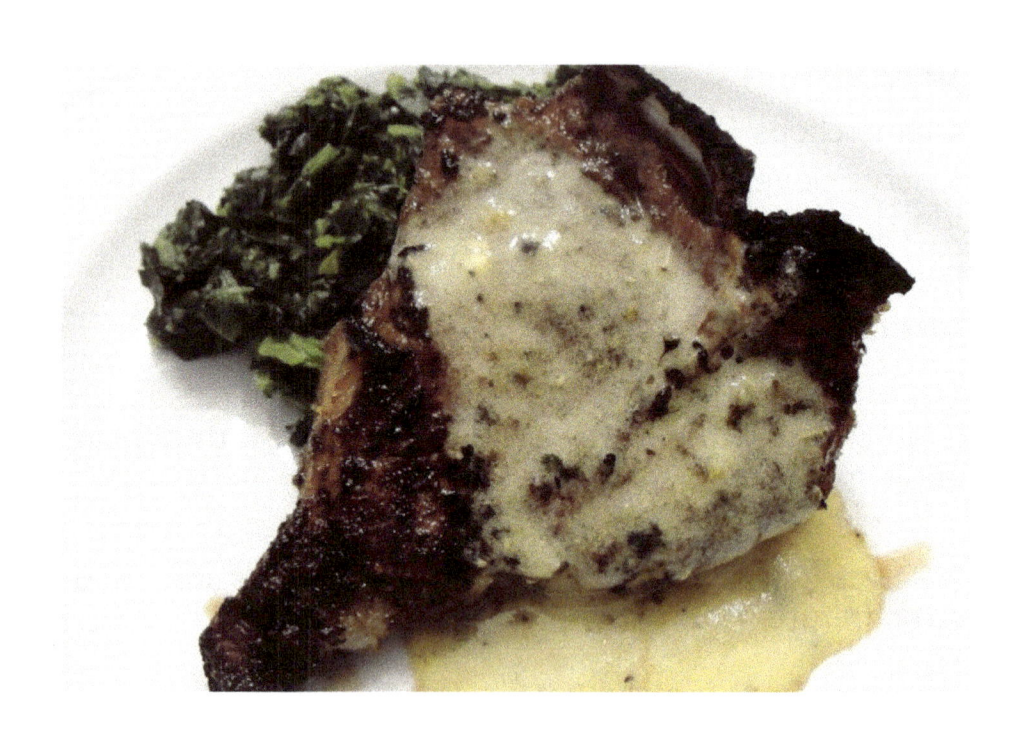

Delicious Herb Beef Patties

Preparation Time:

10 minutes

Cooking Time:

45 minutes

Serve: 4

Ingredients:

10 oz beef minced
1/4 tsp ginger paste
1 1/2 tsp mixed herbs
1 tsp basil
1 tsp tomato puree
1 tsp garlic puree
1/2 tsp mustard
Pepper Salt

Directions:

1.Add all ingredients into the large bowl and mix until well combined. Make patties from meat mixture. Select Air Fry mode.

2.Set time to 45 minutes and temperature 375 F then press START.

3.The air fryer display will prompt you to ADD FOOD once the temperature is reached then place patties in the air fryer basket. Serve and enjoy.

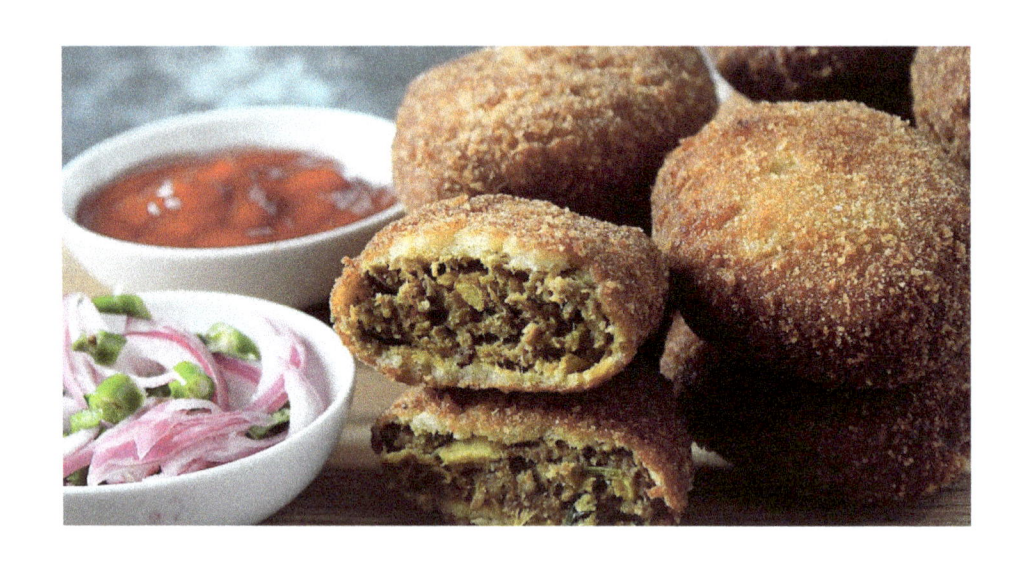

Roasted Sirloin Steak

Preparation Time:

10 minutes

Cooking Time:

30 minutes

Serve: 6

Ingredients:

2 lbs sirloin steak, cut into 1-inch cubes
2 garlic cloves, minced
3 tbsp fresh lemon juice
1 tsp dried oregano
1/4 tsp thyme
1/4 cup water
1/4 cup olive oil
2 cups fresh parsley, chopped
1/2 tsp pepper
1 tsp salt

Directions:

1. Add all ingredients except beef into the large bowl and mix well. Pour bowl mixture into the large zip-lock bag. Add steak cubes into the bag and seal bag and place in refrigerator for 1 hour.

2. Place marinated beef on a baking dish and cover dish with foil. Select Bake mode. Set time to 30 minutes and temperature 400 F then press START.

3. The air fryer display will prompt you to ADD FOOD once the temperature is reached then place the baking

dish in the air fryer basket. Serve and enjoy.

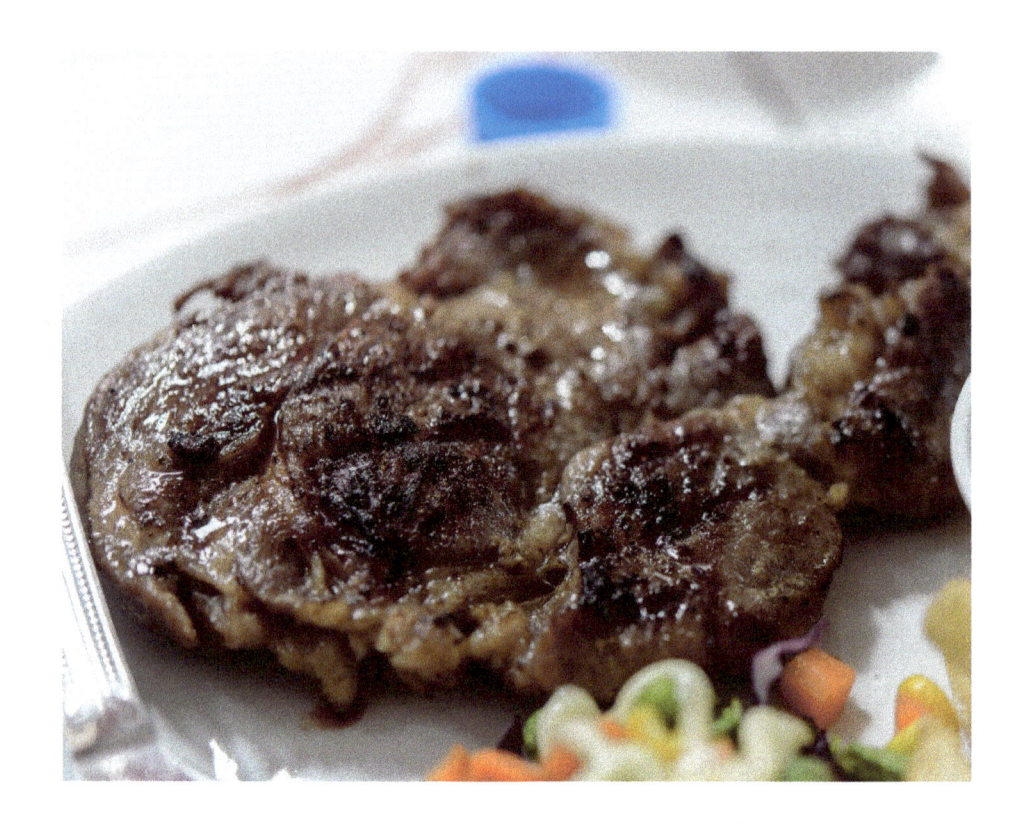

Basil Cheese Lamb Patties

Preparation Time:

10 minutes

Cooking Time:

8 minutes

Serve: 4

Ingredients:

1 lb ground lamb
1 cup goat cheese, crumbled
1 tbsp garlic, minced
6 basil leaves, minced
1 tsp chili powder
1/4 cup mint leaves, minced
1/4 cup fresh parsley, chopped
1 tsp dried oregano
1/4 tsp pepper
1/2 tsp kosher salt

Directions:

1. Add all ingredients into the mixing bowl and mix until well combined. Make four equal shape patties from the meat mixture.

2. Select Bake mode. Set time to 8 minutes and temperature 400 F then press START.

3. The air fryer display will prompt you to ADD FOOD once the temperature is reached then place patties in the air fryer basket. Turn patties halfway through. Serve and enjoy.

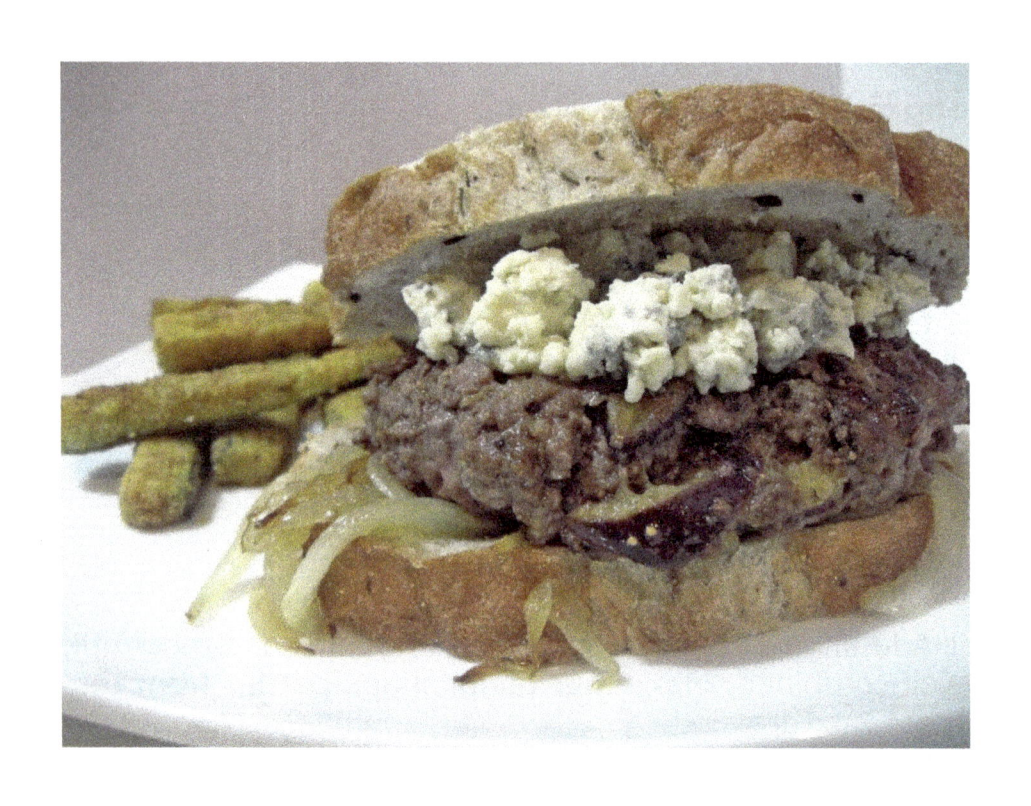

Air Fryer Stew Meat

Preparation Time:

10 minutes

Cooking Time:

25 minutes

Serve: 4

Ingredients:

1 lb beef stew meat, cut into strips
1/2 lime juice
1 tbsp olive oil
1/2 tbsp ground cumin
1 tbsp garlic powder
1/2 tsp onion powder
Pepper Salt

Directions:

Add meat and remaining ingredients into the mixing bowl and mix well. Select Air Fry mode.

2.Set time to 25 minutes and temperature 380 F then press START.

3.The air fryer display will prompt you to ADD FOOD once the temperature is reached then place stew meat in the air fryer basket. Stir halfway through Serve and enjoy.

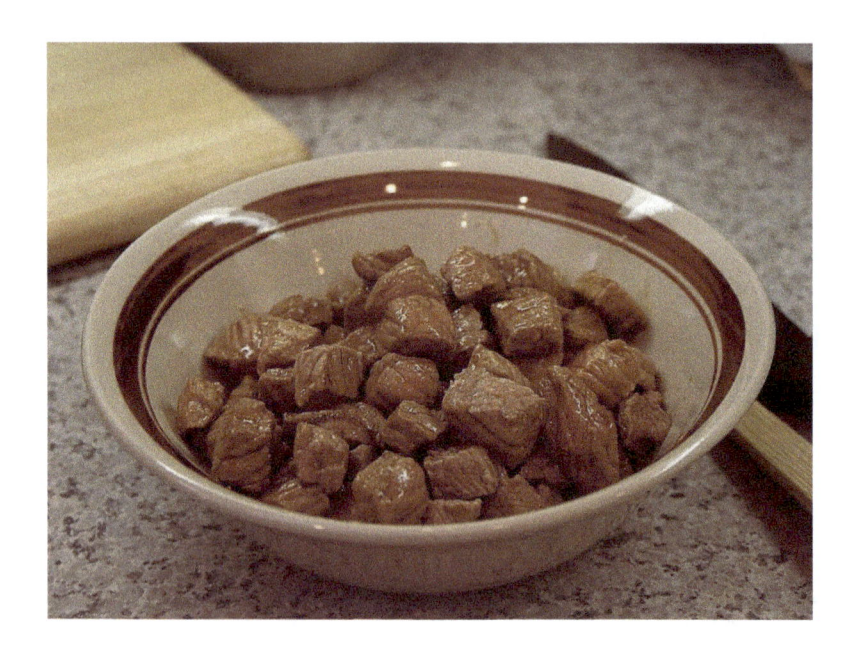

Ranch Pork Chops

Preparation Time:

10 minutes

Cooking Time:

35 minutes

Serve: 4

Ingredients:

4 pork chops, boneless
1 oz ranch seasoning
1 1/2 tbsp olive oil

Directions:

Brush pork chops with oil and rub with ranch seasoning. Select Air Fry mode.

2. Set time to 35 minutes and temperature 400 F then press START.

3. The air fryer display will prompt you to ADD FOOD once the temperature is reached then place pork chops in the air fryer basket. Serve and enjoy.

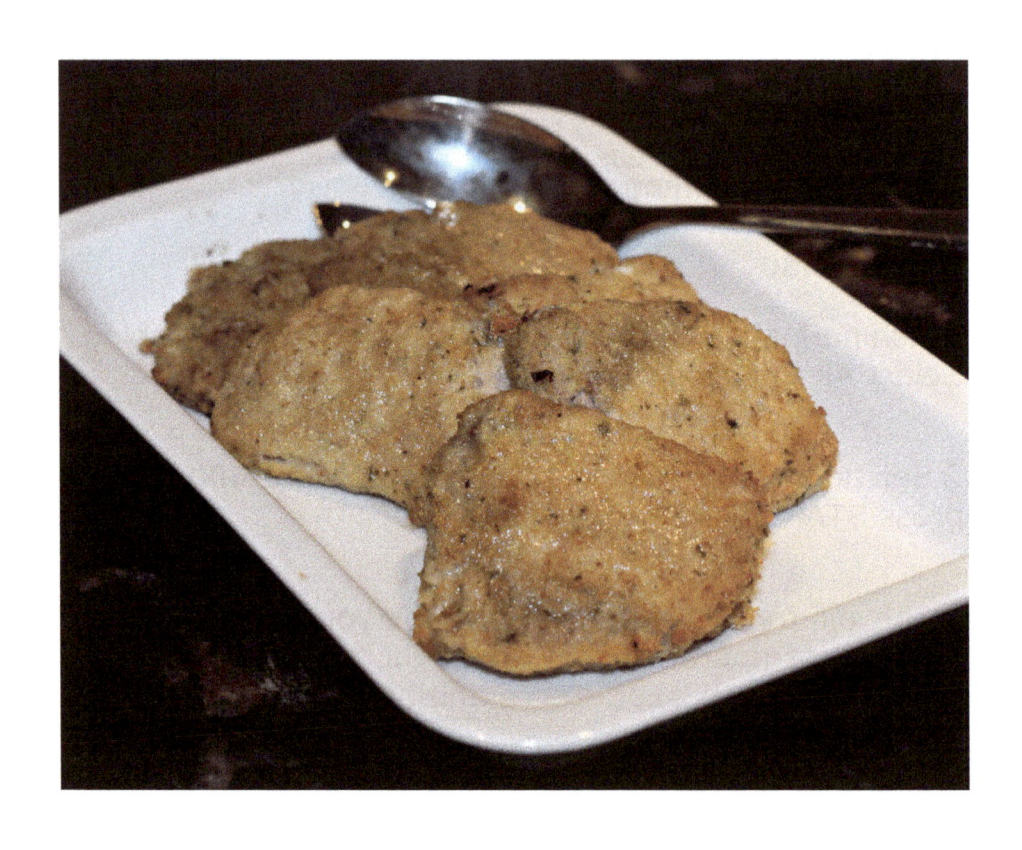

Taco Stuffed Peppers

Preparation Time:

10 minutes

Cooking Time:

8 minutes

Serve: 12

Ingredients:

6 jalapeno peppers, cut in half & remove seeds
1 1/2 tbsp taco seasoning
1/2 lb ground beef
1/4 cup goat cheese, crumbled

Directions:

1. Browned the meat in a large pan. Remove pan from heat. Add taco seasoning to the ground meat and mix well.

2. Stuff meat into each jalapeno half. Select Air Fry mode. Set time to 6 minutes and temperature 320 F then press START.

3. The air fryer display will prompt you to ADD FOOD once the temperature is reached then place jalapeno halves in the air fryer basket. Sprinkle cheese on top of peppers and cook for 2 minutes more. Serve and enjoy.

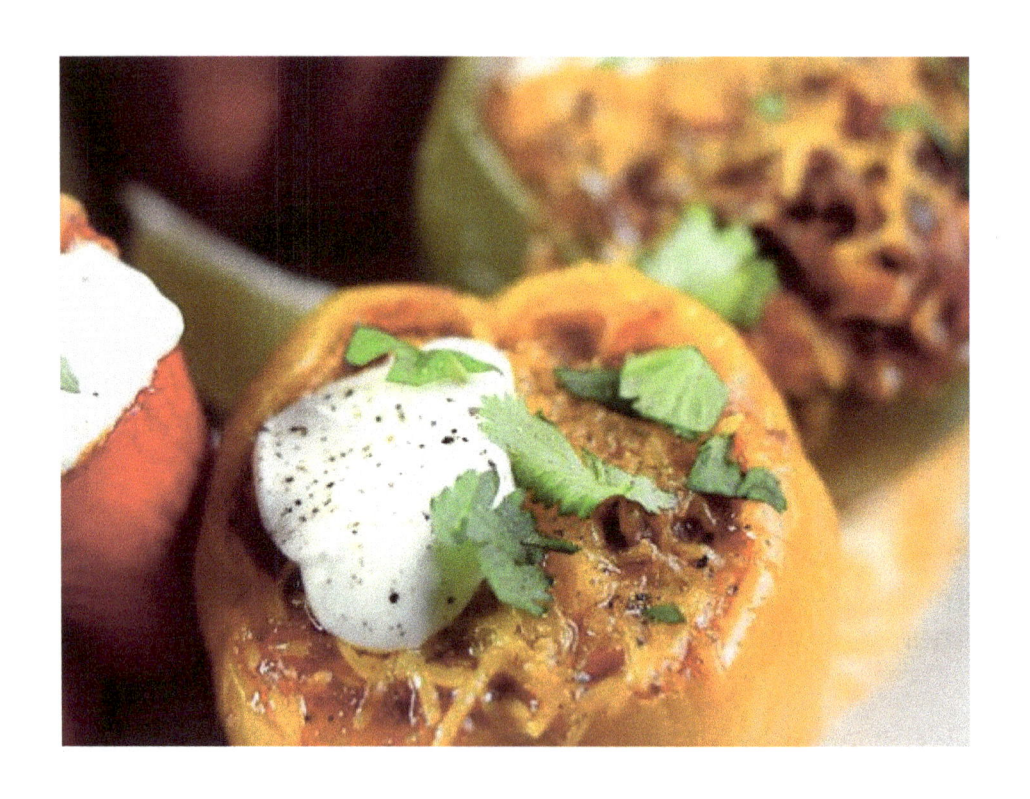

Garlicky Pork Chops

Preparation Time:

10 minutes

Cooking Time:

20 minutes

Serve: 8

Ingredients:

8 pork chops, boneless
6 garlic cloves, minced
1/4 tsp pepper
3/4 cup parmesan cheese
2 tbsp butter, melted
2 tbsp coconut oil
1 tsp thyme
1 tbsp parsley
1/2 tsp sea salt

Directions:

1.In a small bowl, mix together butter, garlic, pepper, thyme, parsley, parmesan cheese, coconut oil, and salt. Brush butter mixture on top of pork chops.

2.Select Air Fry mode. Set time to 20 minutes and temperature 400 F then press START.

3.The air fryer display will prompt you to ADD FOOD once the temperature is reached then place pork chops in the air fryer basket. Turn pork chops halfway through. Serve and enjoy.

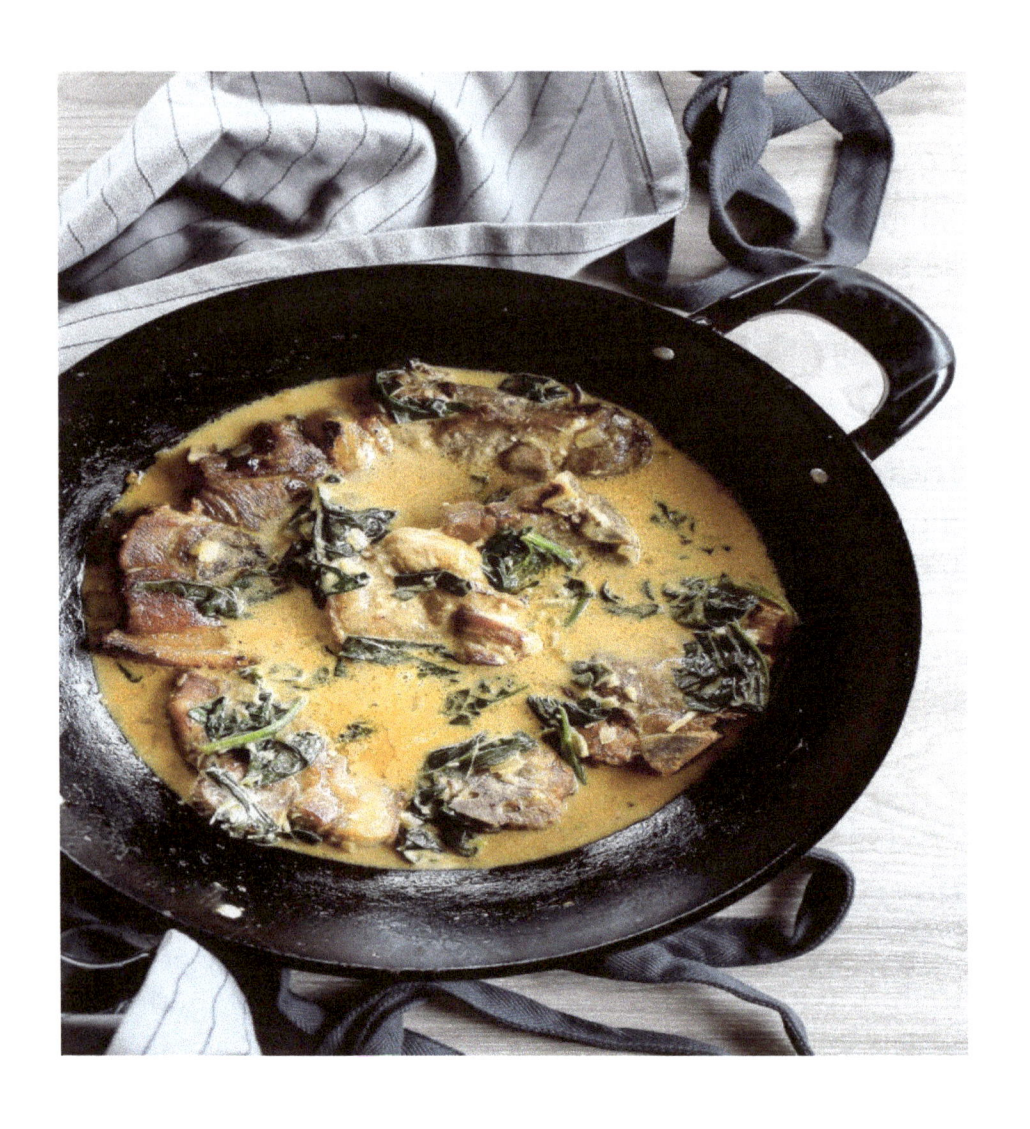

Dijon Pork Chops

Preparation Time:

10 minutes

Cooking Time:

12 minutes

Serve: 4

Ingredients:

4 pork chops
1 tbsp garlic, minced
4 tbsp Dijon mustard
Pepper Salt

Directions:

1. In a small bowl, mix together mustard, garlic, pepper, and salt Brush pork chops with mustard mixture. Select Air Fry mode.

2. Set time to 12 minutes and temperature 350 F then press START.

3. The air fryer display will prompt you to ADD FOOD once the temperature is reached then place pork chops in the air fryer basket. Turn pork chops halfway through. Serve and enjoy.

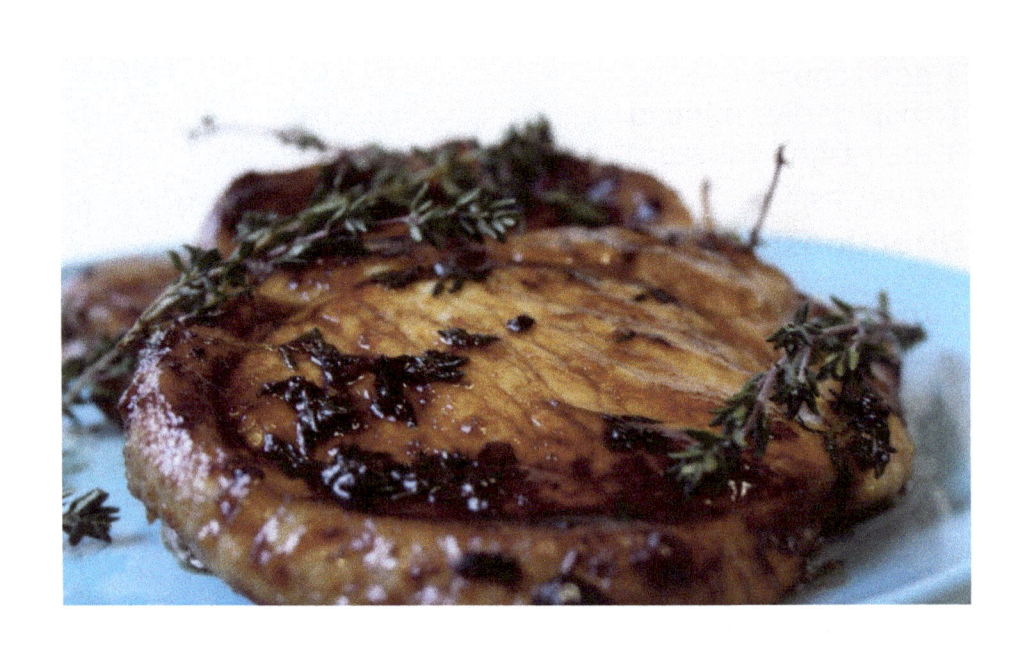

Pecan Dijon Pork Chops

Preparation Time:

10 minutes

Cooking Time:

12 minutes

Serve: 6

Ingredients:

1 egg
6 pork chops, boneless
2 garlic cloves, minced
1 tbsp water
1 tsp Dijon mustard
1 tsp garlic powder
1 tsp onion powder
2 tsp Italian seasoning
1/3 cup arrowroot
1 cup pecans, finely chopped
1/4 tsp salt

Directions:

1. In a shallow bowl, whisk the egg with garlic, water, and Dijon mustard.

2. In a separate shallow bowl, mix together arrowroot, pecans, Italian seasoning, onion powder, garlic powder, and salt.

3.Dip pork chop in the egg mixture and coat with arrowroot mixture. Place the cooking tray in the air fryer basket.

4.Select Air Fry mode. Set time to 12 minutes and temperature 400 F then press START.

5.The air fryer display will prompt you to ADD FOOD once the temperature is reached then place coated pork chops in the air fryer basket.

6.Turn pork chops halfway through. Serve and enjoy.

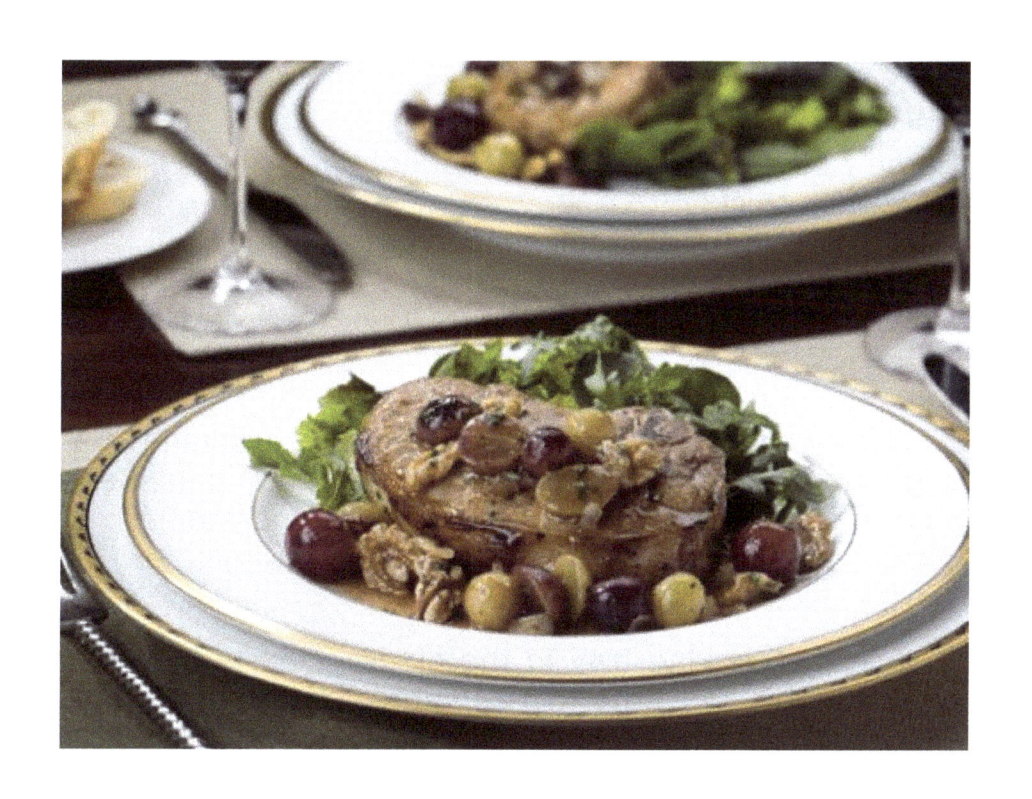

Marinated Ribeye Steaks

Preparation Time:

10 minutes

Cooking Time:

12 minutes

Serve: 4

Ingredients:

1 large ribeye steaks,
1 1/2-inch thick
1 1/2 tbsp Montreal steak seasoning
1/2 cup low-sodium soy sauce
1/4 cup olive oil

Directions:

1. Add soy sauce, oil, and Montreal steak seasoning in a large zip-lock bag. Add steaks in a zip-lock bag. Seal bag shakes well and places in the refrigerator for 2 hours.

2. Place the cooking tray in the air fryer basket. Select Air Fry mode. Set time to 12 minutes and temperature 400 F then press START.

3. The air fryer display will prompt you to ADD FOOD once the temperature is reached then remove steaks from marinade and place in the air fryer basket. Turn steaks halfway through. Serve and enjoy.

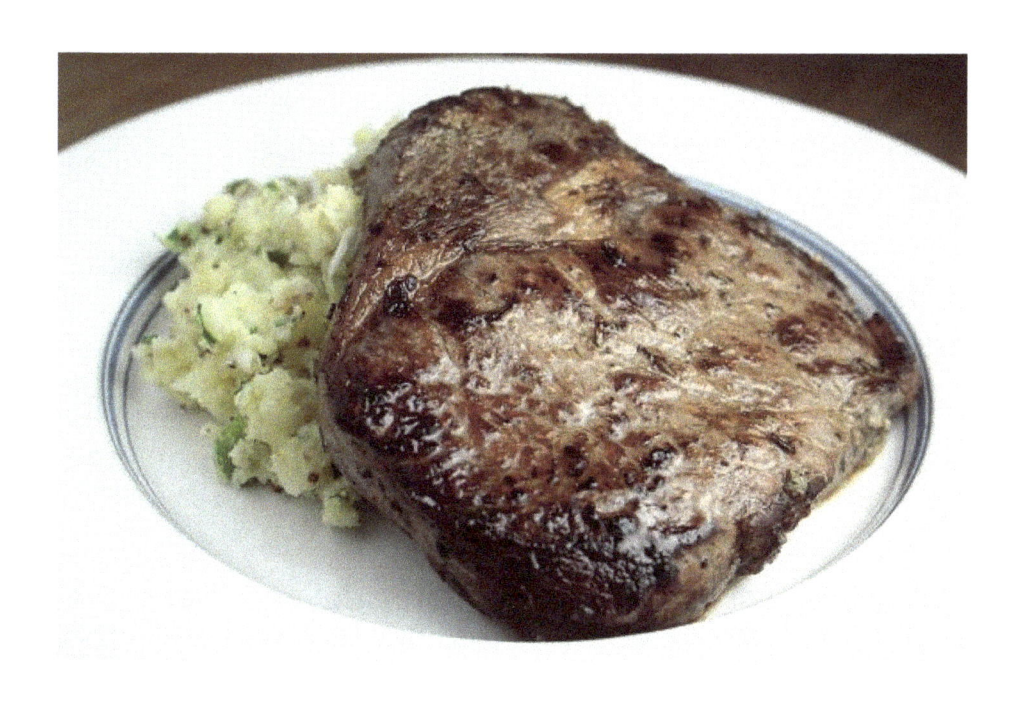

Pork Kebabs

Preparation Time:

10 minutes

Cooking Time:

15 minutes

Serve: 6

Ingredients:

2 lbs country-style pork ribs, cut into cubes
1/4 cup soy sauce
1/2 cup olive oil
1 tbsp Italian seasoning

Directions:

1. Add soy sauce, oil, Italian seasoning, and pork cubes into the zip-lock bag, seal bag and place in the refrigerator for 4 hours.

2. Remove pork cubes from marinade and place the cubes on wooden skewers. Place the cooking tray in the air fryer basket.

3. Line air fryer basket with parchment paper. Select Bake mode.

4. Set time to 15 minutes and temperature 380 F then press START.

5. The air fryer display will prompt you to ADD FOOD

once the temperature is reached then place pork skewers in the air fryer basket. Serve and enjoy

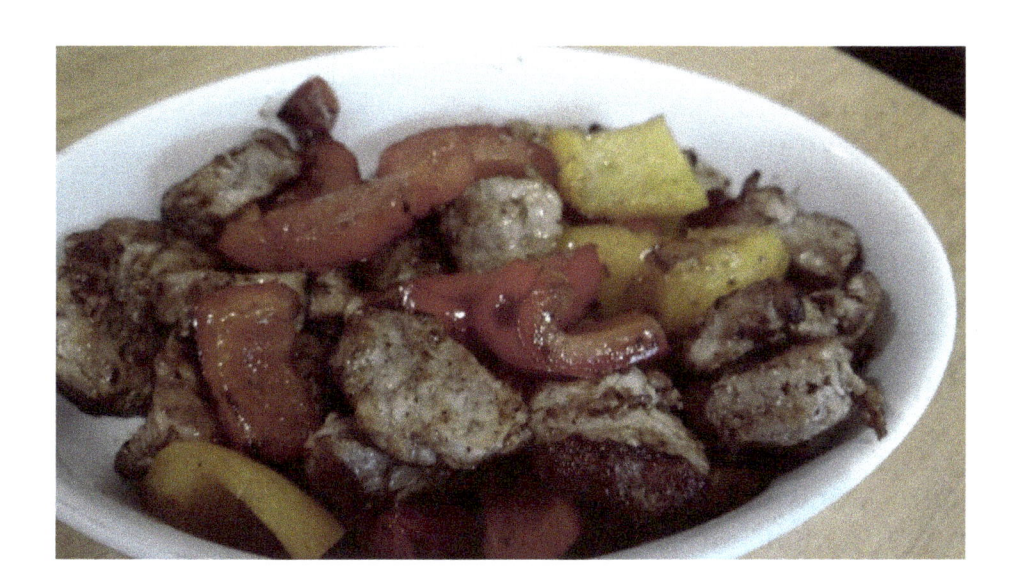

Herb Pork Chops

Preparation Time:

10 minutes

Cooking Time:

15 minutes

Serve: 4

Ingredients:

4 pork chops
2 tsp oregano
2 tsp thyme
2 tsp sage
1 tsp garlic powder
1 tsp paprika
1 tsp rosemary
Pepper Salt

Directions:

1. Spray pork chops with cooking spray. Mix together garlic powder, paprika, rosemary, oregano, thyme, sage, pepper, and salt and rub over pork chops.

2. Select Air Fry mode. Set time to 15 minutes and temperature 360 F then press START.

3. The air fryer display will prompt you to ADD FOOD once the temperature is reached then place pork chops in the air fryer basket.

4. Turn pork chops halfway through. Serve and enjoy.

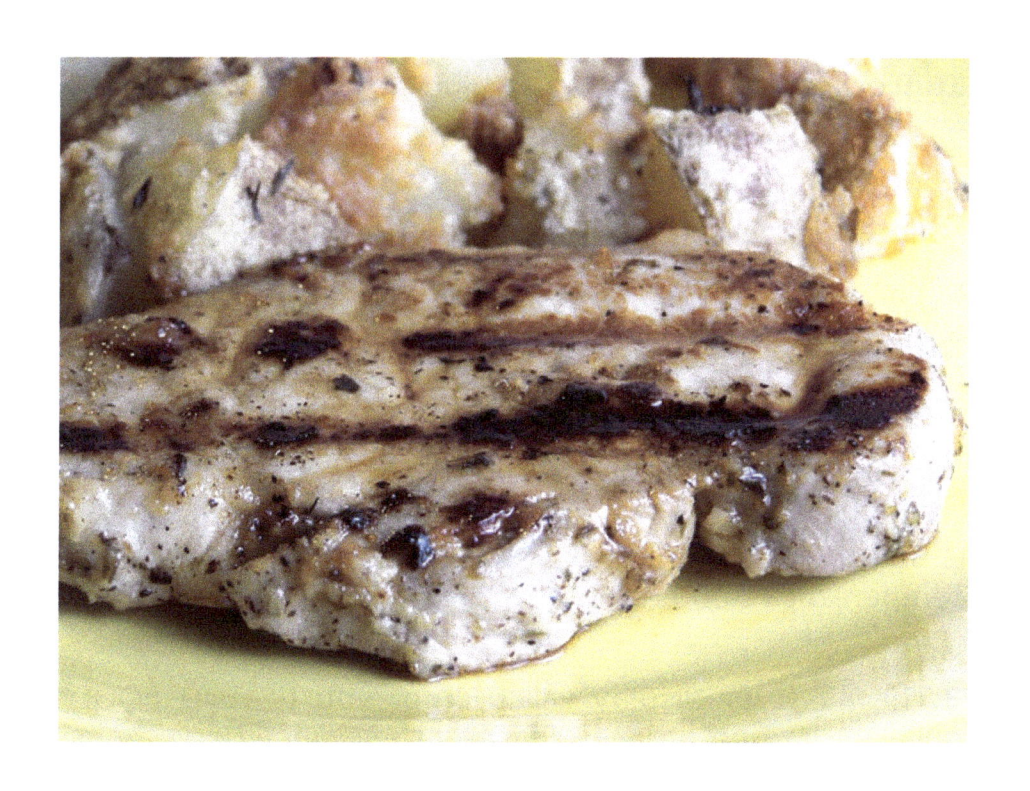

Pork Chops

Preparation Time:

10 minutes

Cooking Time:

14 minutes

Serve: 2

Ingredients:

2 pork chops
1 tsp paprika
1 tsp garlic powder
1 tsp olive oil
Pepper Salt

Directions:

1. Brush pork chops with olive oil and season with garlic powder, paprika, pepper, and salt.

2. Select Air Fry mode. Set time to 14 minutes and temperature 360 F then press START.

3. The air fryer display will prompt you to ADD FOOD once the temperature is reached then place pork chops in the air fryer basket. Turn pork chops halfway through.

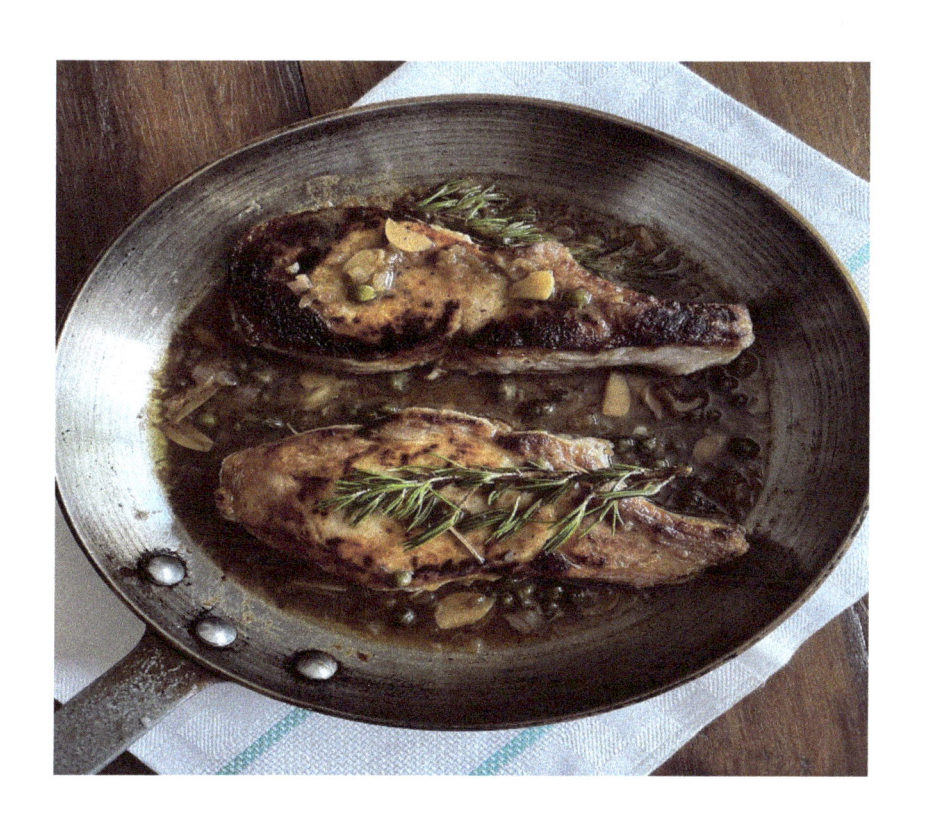

Beef Kebabs

Preparation Time:

10 minutes

Cooking Time:

15 minutes

Serve: 4

Ingredients:

1 lb ground beef
1/2 cup onion, minced
1/4 tsp ground cinnamon
1/4 tsp ground cardamom
1/2 tsp cayenne
1/2 tsp turmeric
1/2 tbsp ginger paste
1/2 tbsp garlic paste
1/4 cup cilantro, chopped
1 tsp salt

Directions:

1. Add meat and remaining ingredients into the large bowl and mix until well combined. Make sausage shape kebabs.

2. Select Bake mode. Set time to 15 minutes and temperature 350 F then press START.

3. The air fryer display will prompt you to ADD FOOD once the temperature is reached then place kebabs in the air fryer basket. Serve and enjoy.

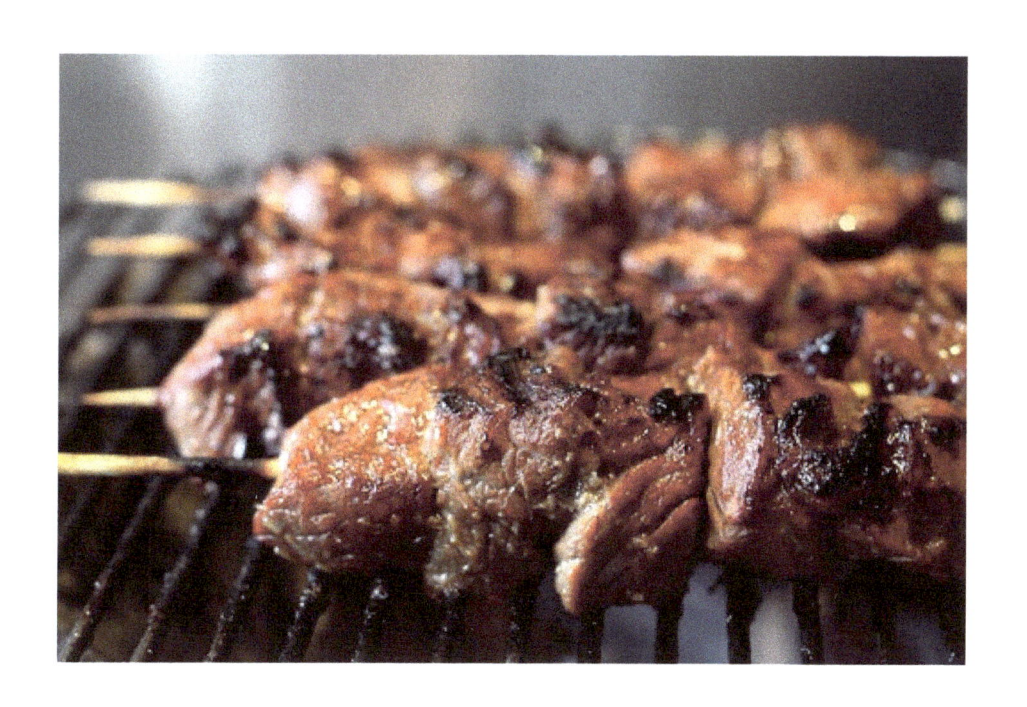

Rosemary Beef Tips

Preparation Time:

10 minutes

Cooking Time:

12 minutes

Serve: 4

Ingredients:

1 lb steak, cut into 1-inch cubes
1 tsp paprika
2 tsp onion powder
1 tsp garlic powder
2 tbsp coconut aminos
2 tsp rosemary, crushed
Pepper Salt

Directions:

1. Add meat and remaining ingredients into the mixing bowl and mix well and let it sit for 5 minutes. Select Air Fry mode.

2. Set time to 12 minutes and temperature 380 F then press START.

3. The air fryer display will prompt you to ADD FOOD once the temperature is reached then place steak cubes in the air fryer basket. Stir halfway through. Serve and enjoy.

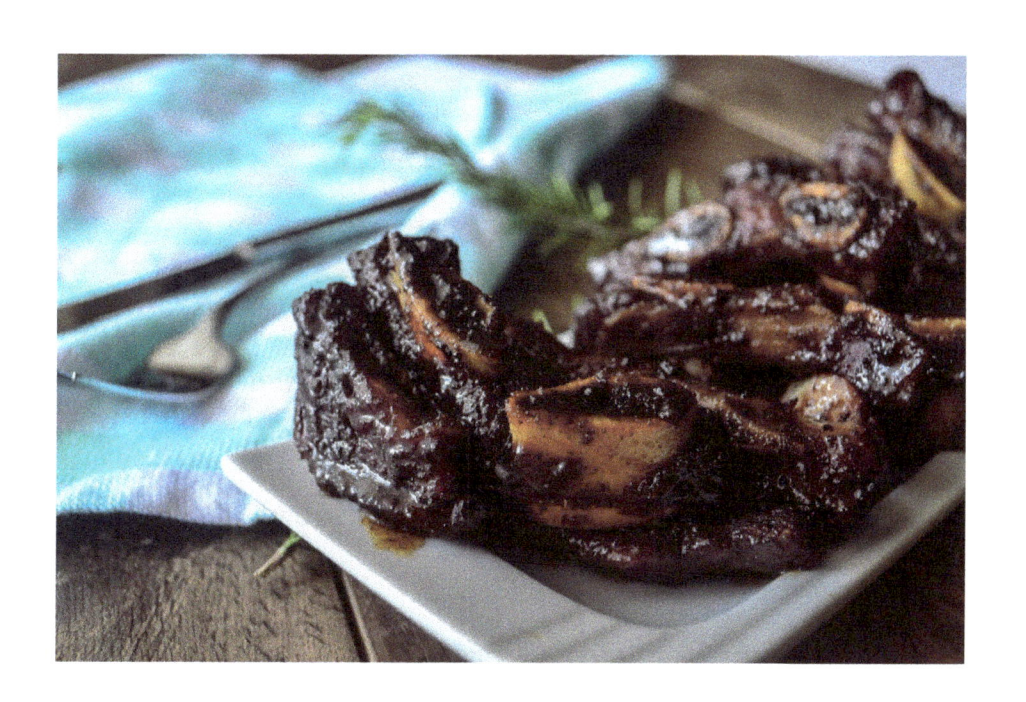

Sirloin Steak

Preparation Time:

10 minutes

Cooking Time:

14 minutes

Serve: 2

Ingredients:

1 lb sirloin steaks
1/2 tsp garlic powder
1/4 tsp onion powder
1 tsp olive oil
Pepper Salt

Directions:

1. Brush steak with olive oil and rub with garlic powder, onion powder, pepper, and salt. Select Air Fry mode.

2. Set time to 14 minutes and temperature 400 F then press START.

3. The air fryer display will prompt you to ADD FOOD once the temperature is reached then place steaks in the air fryer basket. Turn steak halfway through. Serve and enjoy.

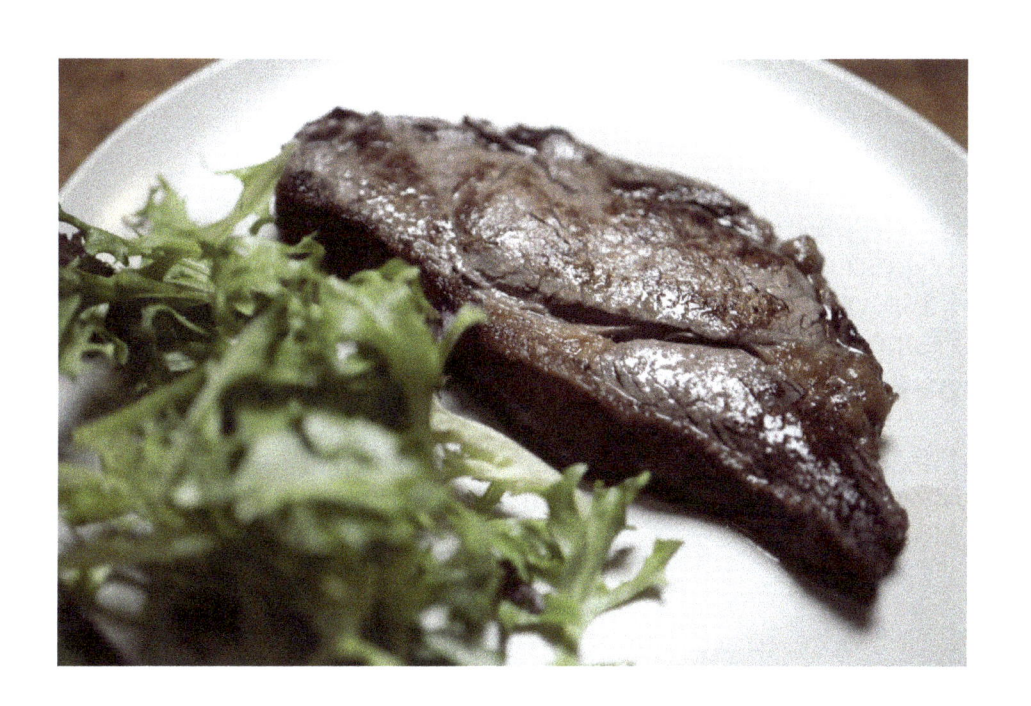

Steak & Mushrooms

Preparation Time:

10 minutes

Cooking Time:

18 minutes

Serve: 4

Ingredients:

1 lb steaks, cut into
1-inch cubes
2 tbsp olive oil
8 oz mushrooms, halved
1/2 tsp garlic powder
1 tsp Worcestershire sauce
Pepper Salt

Directions:

1. Add steak cubes and remaining ingredients into the mixing bowl and toss until well coated. Select Air Fry mode.

2. Set time to 18 minutes and temperature 400 F then press START.

3. The air fryer display will prompt you to ADD FOOD once the temperature is reached then place steak and mushrooms in the air fryer basket.

4. Stir halfway through. Serve and enjoy.

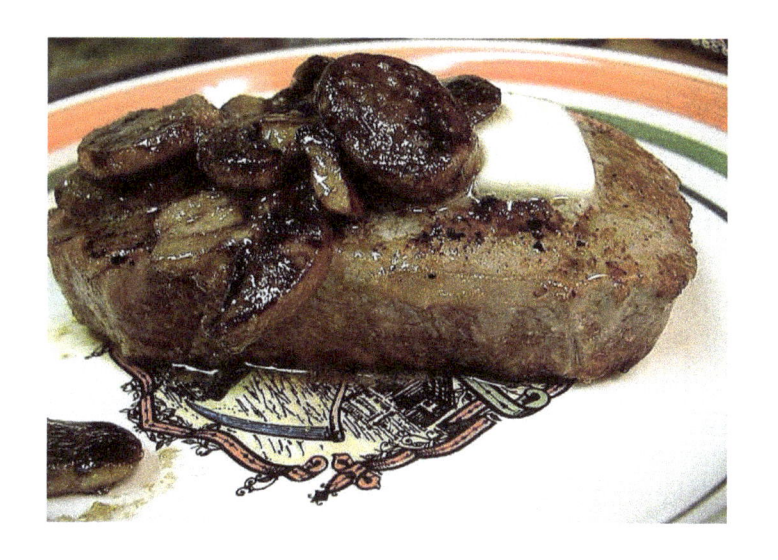

Flavorful Burger Patties

Preparation Time:

10 minutes

Cooking Time:

15 minutes

Serve: 4

Ingredients:

1lb ground lamb
1/4 tsp cayenne pepper
1/4 cup fresh parsley, chopped
1/4 cup onion, minced
1 tbsp garlic, minced
1/2 tsp ground allspice
1 tsp ground cinnamon
1 tsp ground coriander
1 tsp ground cumin
1/4 tsp pepper
1 tsp kosher salt

Directions:

1. Add all ingredients into the large bowl and mix until well combined.

2. Make 4 patties from the meat mixture. Select Bake mode. Set time to 14 minutes and temperature 375 F then press START.

3. The air fryer display will prompt you to ADD FOOD once the temperature is reached then place patties in the air fryer basket.

4.Turn patties halfway through. Serve and enjoy

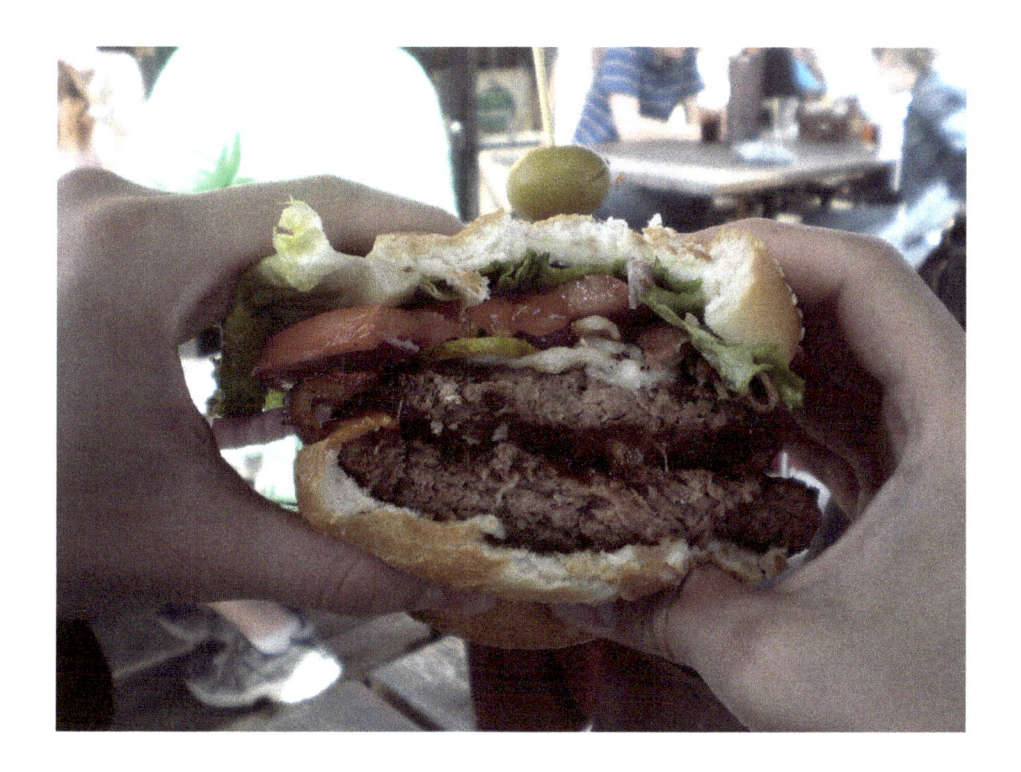

Baked Beef & Broccoli

Preparation Time:

10 minutes

Cooking Time:

25 minutes

Serve: 2

Ingredients:

1/2 cup broccoli florets
1/2 lb beef stew meat, cut into pieces
1 onion, sliced
1 tbsp vinegar
1 tbsp olive oil
Pepper Salt

Directions:

1. Add meat and remaining ingredients into the large bowl and toss well.

2. Select Bake mode. Set time to 25 minutes and temperature 390 F then press START.

3. The air fryer display will prompt you to ADD FOOD once the temperature is reached then place beef and broccoli in the air fryer basket. Serve and enjoy.

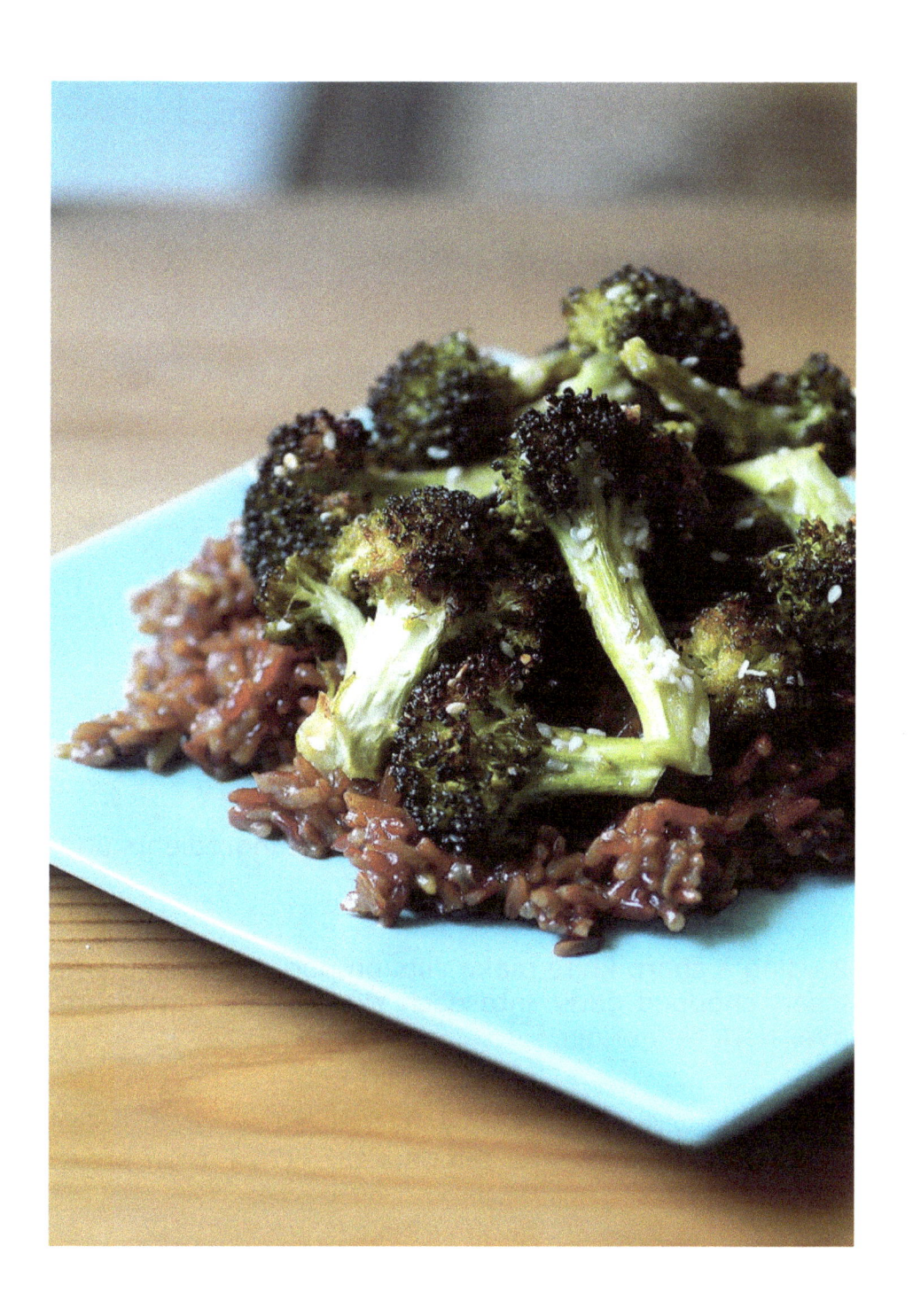

Spiced Pork Tenderloin

Preparation Time:

10 minutes

Cooking Time:

35 minutes

Serve: 6

Ingredients:

1lbs pork tenderloin
For the spice mix:
1/2 tsp allspice
1 tsp cinnamon
1 tsp cumin
1 tsp coriander
1/4 tsp cayenne
1 tsp oregano
1/4 tsp cloves

Directions:

1.In a small bowl, mix together all spice ingredients and set aside.

2.Using a sharp knife make slits on pork tenderloin and insert chopped garlic into each slit. Rub spice mixture over pork tenderloin.

3.Sprinkle with pepper and salt. Select Bake mode. Set time to 35 minutes and temperature 375 F then press START.

4.The air fryer display will prompt you to ADD FOOD once the temperature is reached then place pork tenderloin in the air fryer basket. Serve and enjoy.

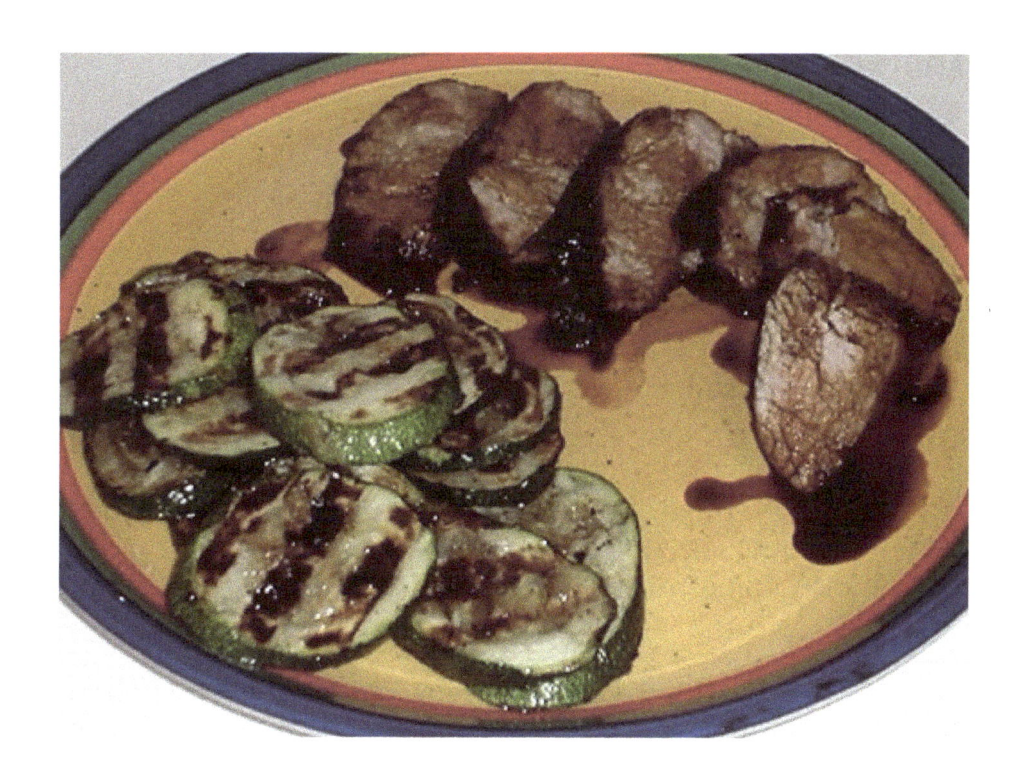

Spicy Pork Chops

Preparation Time:

10 minutes

Cooking Time:

10 minutes

Serve: 4

Ingredients:

4 pork chops
1/2 tsp black pepper
1/2 tsp ground cumin
1 1/2 tsp olive oil
1/2 tsp dried sage
1 tsp cayenne pepper
1 tsp paprika
1/2 tsp garlic salt

Directions:

1. In a small bowl, mix together paprika, garlic salt, sage, pepper, cayenne pepper, and cumin. Rub pork chops with spice mixture.

2. Spray pork chops with cooking spray. Select Bake mode. Set time to 10 minutes and temperature 400 F then press START.

3. The air fryer display will prompt you to ADD FOOD once the temperature is reached then place pork chops in the air fryer basket.

4. Turn pork chops halfway through. Serve and enjoy.

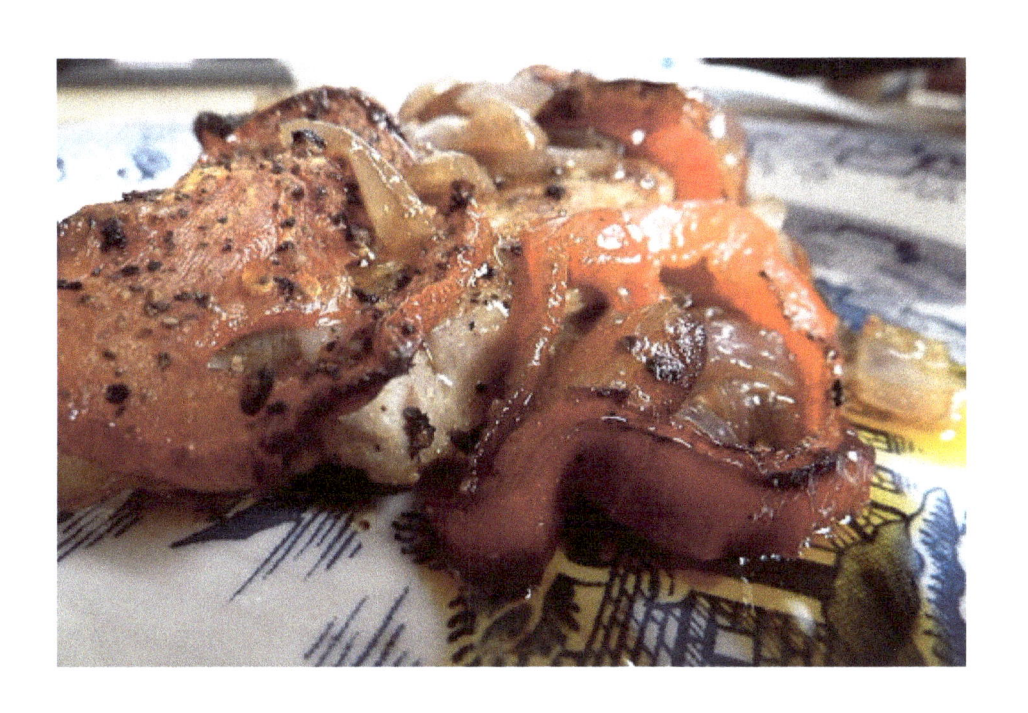

Lemon Herb Lamb Chops

Preparation Time:

10 minutes

Cooking Time:

16 minutes

Serve: 4

Ingredients:

1lb lamb chops
1 tsp coriander
1 tsp oregano
1 tsp thyme
1 tsp rosemary
2 tbsp fresh lemon juice
2 tbsp olive oil
1 tsp salt

Directions:

1. Add all ingredients except lamb chops into the zip-lock bag.

2. Add lamb chops to the bag. Seal bag and place in the refrigerator overnight.

3. Select Air Fry mode. Set time to 16 minutes and temperature 390 F then press START.

3. The air fryer display will prompt you to ADD FOOD once the temperature is reached then place lamb chops in the air fryer basket.

4.Turn lamb chops halfway through. Serve and enjoy.

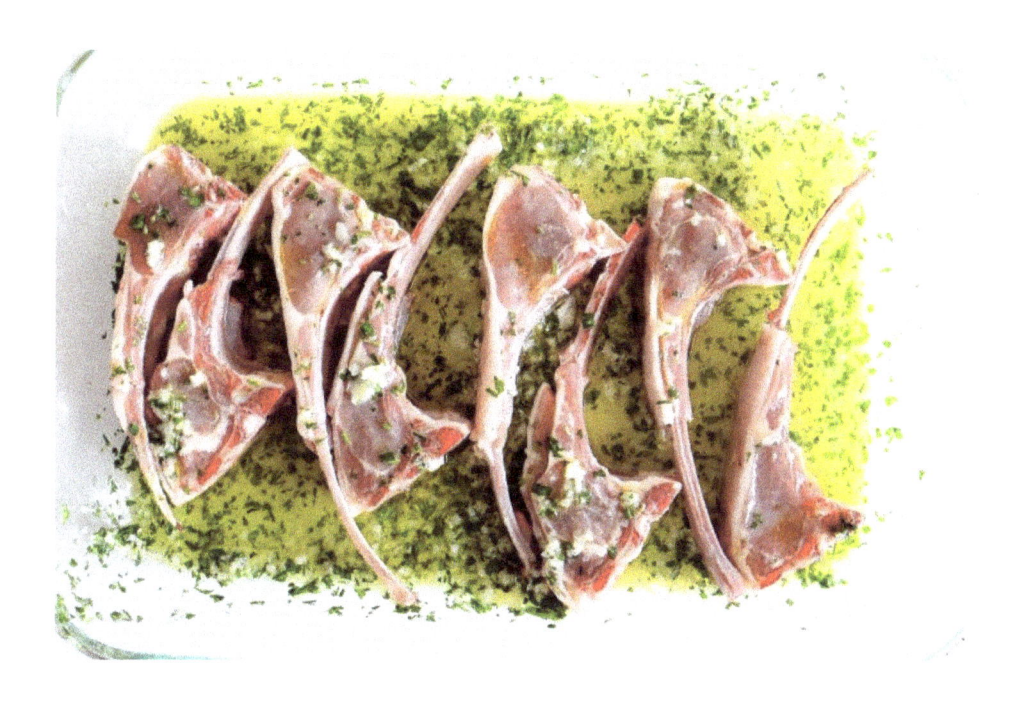

Cajun Herb Pork Chops

Preparation Time:

10 minutes

Cooking Time:

9 minutes

Serve: 2

Ingredients:

1 pork chops, boneless
1 tsp herb de Provence
1 tsp paprika
1/2 tsp Cajun seasoning
3 tbsp parmesan cheese, grated
1/3 cup almond flour

Directions:

1. Mix together almond flour, Cajun seasoning, herb de Provence, paprika, and parmesan cheese. Spray both the pork chops with cooking spray.

2. Coat both the pork chops with almond flour mixture. Select Bake mode.

3. Set time to 8 minutes and temperature 350 F then press START.

4. The air fryer display will prompt you to ADD FOOD once the temperature is reached then place pork chops in the air fryer basket.

5.Turn pork chops halfway through. Serve and enjoy.

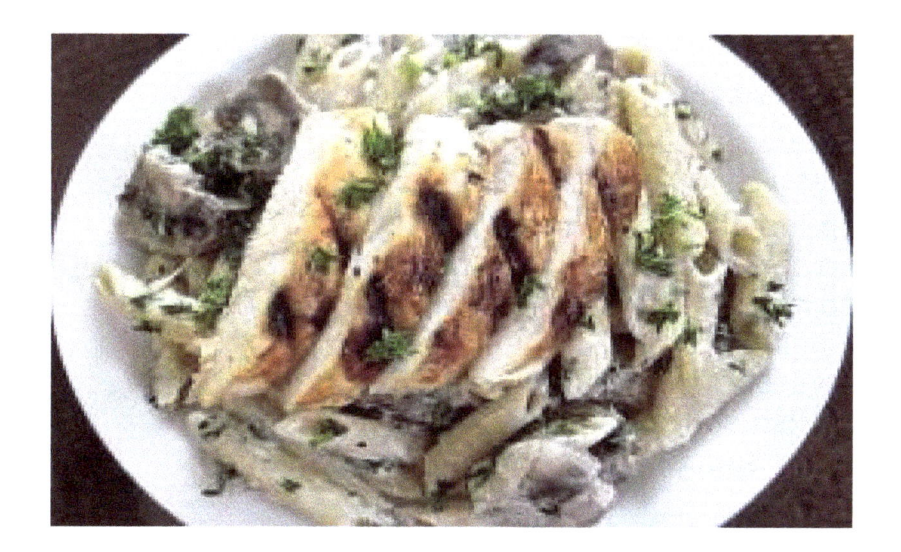

Thai Pork Chops

Preparation Time:

10 minutes

Cooking Time:

12 minutes

Serve: 2

Ingredients:

1.2 pork chops
1 tsp black pepper
3 tbsp lemongrass, chopped
1 tbsp shallot, chopped
1 tbsp garlic, chopped
1 tsp liquid stevia
1 tbsp sesame oil
1 tbsp fish sauce
1 tsp soy sauce

Directions:

1.Add pork chops in a mixing bowl. Pour remaining ingredients over the pork chops and mix well.

2.Place in refrigerator for 2 hours. Select Air Fry mode. Set time to 12 minutes and temperature 400 F then press START.

3.The air fryer display will prompt you to ADD FOOD once the temperature is reached then place marinated pork chops in the air fryer basket. Serve and enjoy.

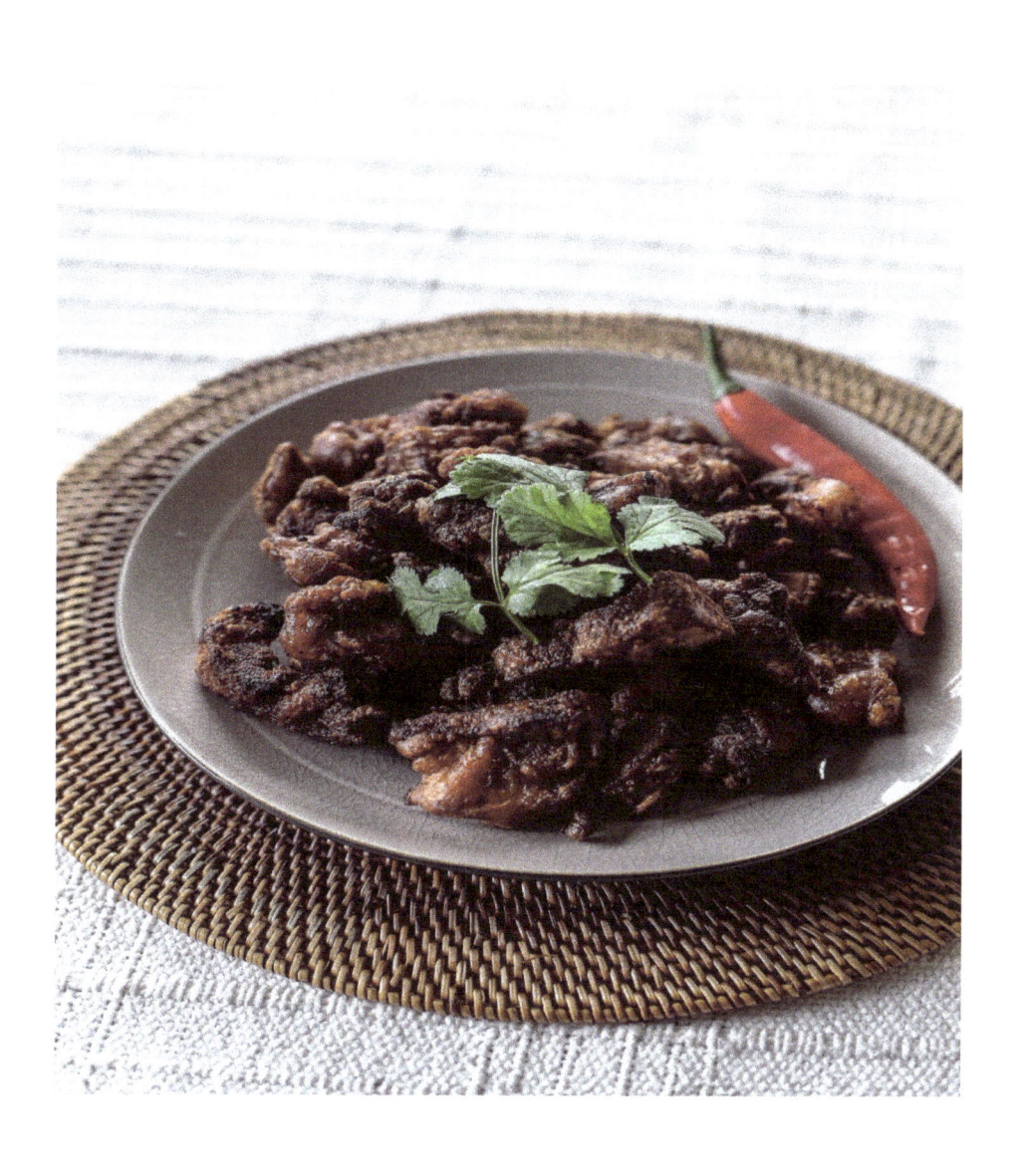

Spicy Asian Lamb

Preparation Time:

10 minutes

Cooking Time:

10 minutes

Serve: 4

Ingredients:

1 lb lamb, cut into 2-inch pieces
1 tbsp soy sauce
2 tbsp vegetable oil
1/2 tsp cayenne
1 1/2 tbsp ground cumin
1/4 tsp liquid stevia
2 red chili peppers, chopped
1 tbsp garlic, minced
1 tsp salt

Directions:

1. Mix together cumin and cayenne in a small bowl. Rub meat with cumin mixture and place in a large bowl.

2. Add oil, soy sauce, garlic, chili peppers, stevia, and salt over the meat. Mix well and place in the refrigerator overnight.

3. Select Air Fry mode. Set time to 10 minutes and temperature 360 F then press START.

4.The air fryer display will prompt you to ADD FOOD once the temperature is reached then place marinated meat in the air fryer basket. Serve and enjoy.

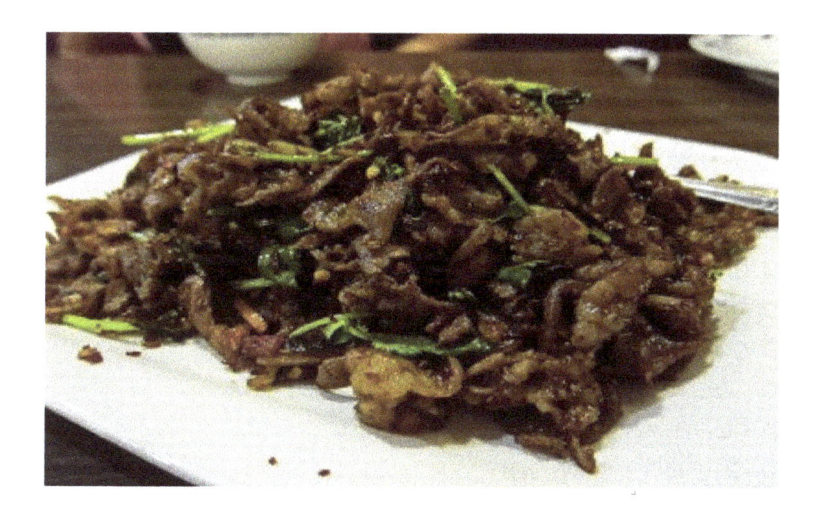

Chipotle Steak

Preparation Time:

10 minutes

Cooking Time:

10 minutes

Serve: 3

Ingredients:

1 lb ribeye steak
1/4 tsp onion powder
1/4 tsp garlic powder
1/4 tsp chili powder
1/2 tsp black pepper
1/2 tsp coffee powder
1/8 tsp cocoa powder
1/8 tsp coriander powder
1/4 tsp chipotle powder
1/4 tsp paprika
1 1/2 tsp sea salt

Directions:

1. In a small bowl, mix together all ingredients except steak.

2. Rub spice mixture all over the steak and let sit the steak for 30 minutes.

3. Select Air Fry mode. Set time to 10 minutes and temperature 390 F then press START.

4.The air fryer display will prompt you to ADD FOOD once the temperature is reached then place steak in the air fryer basket. Turn steak halfway through. Serve and enjoy.

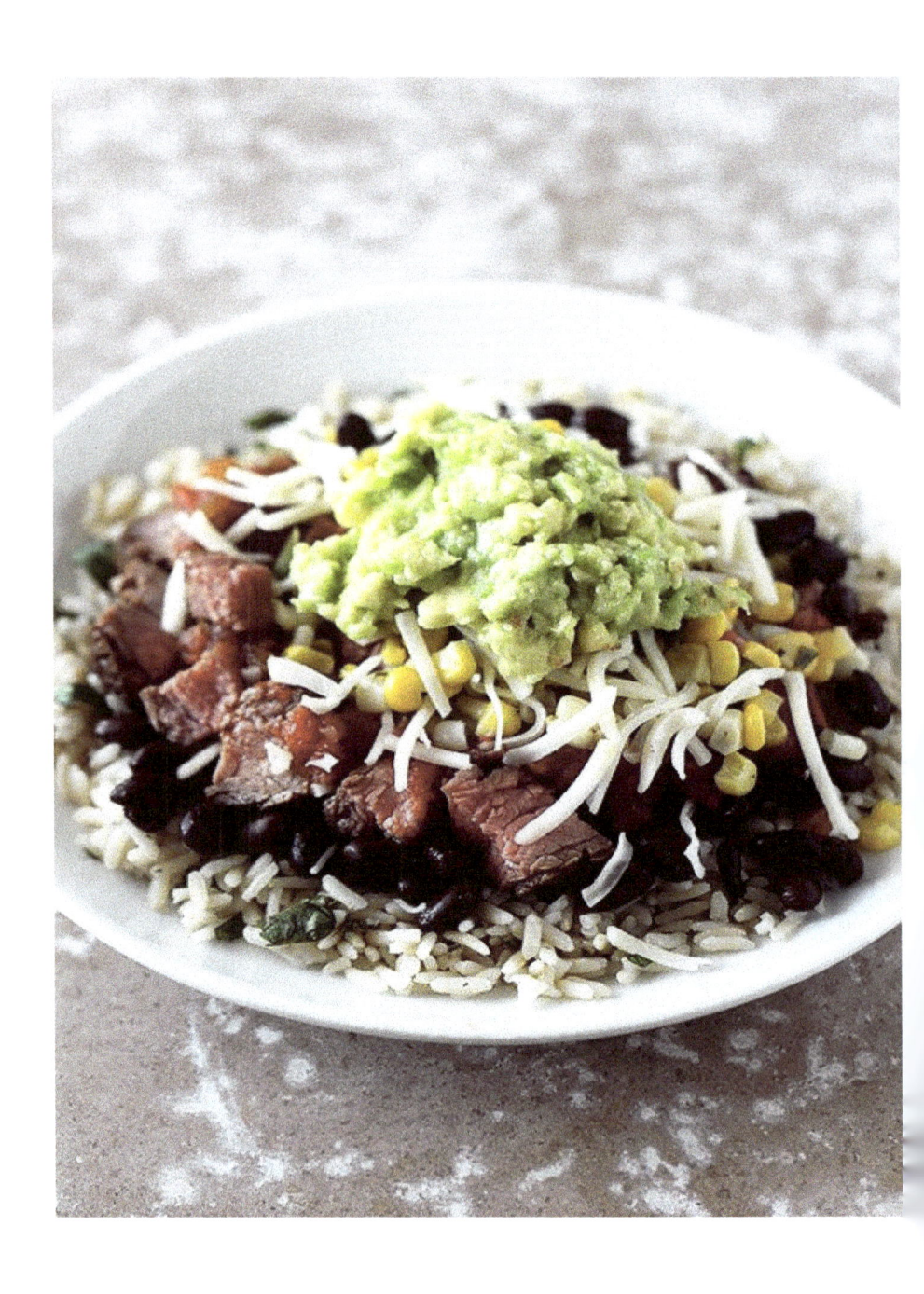

Lightning Source UK Ltd.
Milton Keynes UK
UKHW021022220922
409258UK00001B/14

9 781802 691641